40/4
-91

Bull's-Eye

Bull's-Eye

Unraveling the Medical Mystery of Lyme Disease

SECOND EDITION

Jonathan A. Edlow, M.D.

Yale University Press

New Haven and London

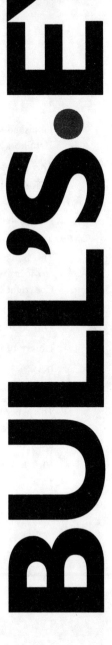

BULL'S·EYE

Published with assistance from the foundation established in memory of Philip Hamilton McMillan of the Class of 1894, Yale College.

This Second Edition published 2004 by Yale University Press
First Edition published 2003 by Yale University Press

Printed in the United States of America

Library of Congress Control Number: 2003116746

ISBN 0-300-10370-0 (pbk. : alk. paper)

A catalogue record for this book is available from the British Library.

The paper in this book meets the guidelines for permanence and durability of the Committee on Production Guidelines for Book Longevity of the Council on Library Resources.

10 9 8 7 6 5 4 3 2 1

To the memory of my mother, Bernice Amernick Edlow,
who, both by her encouragement and her example,
first instilled in me the love of books and of reading.

"The philosophies of one age have become the absurdities of the next, and the foolishness of yesterday has become the wisdom of tomorrow."
—Sir William Osler

"The radical invents the views. When he has worn them out, the conservative adopts them."
—Mark Twain

"Discovery consists in seeing what everyone else has seen and thinking what no one else has thought."
—Albert Szent-Gyorgi

"It is a capital mistake to theorize before you have all the evidence. It biases the judgment."
—Sherlock Holmes in *A Study in Scarlet*, Arthur Conan Doyle

CONTENTS

Preface to the Second Edition ix

Preface xiii

Acknowledgments xvi

Chronology xviii

1 A Family Under Siege 1

2 A Little Girl's Knee 9

3 The Broad Street Pump 17

4 An Appointment in New Haven 28

5 An Outbreak of Arthritis 36

6 An Outbreak of Dermatitis 46

7 The European Connection 55

8 Further Work in Europe 62

9 The Blind Men and the Elephant 72

10 The Connection with Ticks 81

11 An Intersection of Investigations 90

12 From the Alps to the Rockies 102

13 To Treat or Not to Treat? 110

14 The Scramble for the Cause 118

15 The Culmination of Efforts 130

16 Progress to the End of the 1980s 141

17 A Geographical Expansion 150

18 The Diagnostician's Dilemma 160

19 Ambiguity in the Lab 170

20 A Tick with Two Toxins 179

21 Cracks in the Theory 188

22 Another Paradigm 199

23 Therapeutic Adventures 212

24 Genomes and Vaccines 221

25 Legal and Political Battles 231

26 An Independent Reality 243

Epilogue 251

Appendix 255

   A: Symptoms of Lyme Disease 255

   B: Tick-Borne Diseases in Humans and Animals 256

Sources 259

Glossary 275

Index 279

The hardcover version of this book was on the shelves of bookstores for only five months when I was asked to write a preface for the paperback edition. I had penned the preface for the original book just one year before. In it I wrote, "Undoubtedly, some people from both sides of this divide will feel that I have misstated their positions. If so, perhaps this will be a mark of success."

As I predicted, *Bull's Eye* has elicited mixed reactions among the opposing groups of people who feel strongly about Lyme disease. Many of the reviews and responses I received were flattering; others were quite the opposite. Although I had taken great pains to present a balanced view of the controversial issues surrounding Lyme disease, some readers took umbrage. People aligned with the "conventional" camp have charged that by presenting the "alternative" viewpoint side by side with the conventional, I gave the alternative camp too much credibility. Some from the alternative camp believed that I unfairly boosted the conventional side and avoided showing the human dimension of the conflict. I am not in a position to respond to these critiques dispassionately. Yet the fact that they came from both camps suggests that I did succeed in presenting both points of view.

Although I anticipated the controversy, I did not predict the large volume of telephone calls and letters that I received from readers throughout the United States—people who were suffering from various chronic symptoms and who believed that they had Lyme disease. I am sure that some of them did have Lyme disease and equally certain that others did not. Not having examined them or their medical records, I have no way of knowing which patients fall into which category. But the phone conversations were moving and also, I think, telling. The callers felt disconnected from the medical profession; their needs were going unmet. There are, I believe, two reasons for this. First, the current medical-economic climate increasingly translates patient interactions into the language of minutes and dollars. Physicians do not have sufficient time to listen, be curious, and explore. Second, the medical-political climate discourages alternative points of view, especially with respect to the controversial aspects of Lyme disease. Thus many physicians simply do not want to deal with the hassle of treating patients who think they have Lyme disease or of fighting City Hall to support their medical policies.

One physician who does is Dr. Joseph Burrascano Jr., who at the time that I finished writing the first edition was embroiled in a legal quagmire with the Office of Professional Medical Conduct (OPMC) at the New York State Department of Health. In a mixed decision the board found misconduct on some charges and lack of misconduct on others. In its final report, the committee wrote,

> The Hearing Committee recognizes the existence of the current debate within the medical community over issues concerning management of patients with recurrent or long term Lyme disease. This appears to be a highly polarized and politicized conflict, as was demonstrated to this committee by expert testimony from both sides, each supported by numerous medical journal articles, and each emphatic that the opposite position was clearly incorrect. In fact, it often appeared that the testimony was framed to espouse specific viewpoints, rather than directly answer questions posed. What clearly did emerge however was that the Respondent's [Burrascano's] approach, while certainly a minority viewpoint, is one that is shared by many other physicians. We recognize that the practice of medicine may not always be an exact science, "issued guidelines" are not regulatory, and patient care is frequently individualized.
>
> We are also acutely aware that it was not this Committee's role to resolve this medical debate, but rather to answer the questions raised in the statement of charges. . . .
>
> The Hearing Committee has fully reviewed the full range of penalties available, from censure to revocation. It is our carefully considered decision that the Respondent should be suspended from the practice of medicine for six months, with the entire period of suspension stayed. During that period, the Respondent shall be on probation, under the supervision of a practice monitor, who is board certified in infectious diseases.

One may interpret this result as one chooses. The Foundation for Advancement of Innovative Medicine chose to claim, on its Web site, that Dr. Burrascano has been "exonerated." On the OPMC Web site, he is listed as "guilty of negligence on more than one occasion." It is worth noting that Dr. Burrascano's patients strongly supported him throughout this ordeal.

To what degree the truth is muddied by politics is difficult to know. But it is abundantly clear that these same politics continue to color both sides' interpretation of facts.

Since the first edition of this book appeared, there have been only a few scientific advances, but some interesting new studies have been published. And it should come as no surprise that some of them are mired in controversy. An article published in the *Annals of Internal Medicine* (Gary P. Wormser and colleagues, "Duration of Antibiotic Therapy for Early Lyme Disease," May 2003) expanded on data reported at the Ninth International Conference on Lyme Borreliosis and Other Tick-Borne Diseases (August 2002). The authors of this article suggested that ten days of therapy, rather than the more usual fourteen to twenty-one days, were sufficient to treat erythema migrans, the rash of early Lyme disease. The study was designed to be beyond reproach—a randomized, double-blind, placebo-controlled protocol. Yet its results were soon challenged.

Dr. Andrea Gaito, president of the International Lyme and Associated Diseases Society (ILADS), writes on its Web site (accessed October 2, 2003), "The article entitled 'Duration of Antibiotic Therapy for Early Lyme Disease' recently published in the Annals of Internal Medicine is flawed in its methodology and its findings. The collective experience of ILADS physicians has shown that 10 days of therapy has consistently proven insufficient in preventing the development of systemic manifestations of Lyme disease. Our experience proves most patients who are treated with short duration antibiotics return for repeat therapy when their symptoms do not improve." Other position statements on the Web site argue against the Centers for Disease Control and Prevention diagnostic criteria and the mainstream position that long-term antibiotics are unnecessary for treating Lyme disease.

The link between *Bartonella* (a group of bacterial species, one of which is associated with cat-scratch fever) and Lyme disease is tantalizing. *Bartonella* clearly are found in ticks that bite humans. However, their connection to ongoing symptoms following treatment for Lyme disease remains to be fully elucidated. In 2003, *Bartonella* species were found on human-biting ticks in Italy.

In other international news, new *Borrelia* species have been found in Turkey. Some of these have been of the relapsing fever variety, but *B. burgdorferi*, the causative agent of Lyme disease, has also been found.

Now that the first Lyme disease vaccine, using the protein Osp A, has been pulled from the market, research groups are investigating other candidate vaccines. One German group found that an OspC sequence was successful in inducing a strong protective antibody response in mice. Human trials, however, are a long way off.

Many other small bits of research and experimental data from scientists and laboratories across the globe continue to be reported. The march toward better understanding of this complex infection continues, but only one step at a time, and with occasional missteps. For now, our collective understanding of Lyme disease remains a perfect example of the kind of paradigm shift that Thomas Kuhn described—with both sides talking, but not to each other.

When I attended medical school at the University of Maryland from 1974 to 1978, Lyme disease was not part of the curriculum. In fact, the term had not even been coined yet. The first publications about this phenomenon were just beginning to make their way into the medical literature, and the etiology had not been discovered. Most U.S. physicians had never heard of Lyme disease, and those who had were not recommending antibiotics for treatment. The presumptive cause, after all, was a virus; the notion that the disease was related to ticks was still just conjecture.

Other diseases transmitted by tick bite were on the wane in the United States and also did not occupy much time in the curriculum. The chairman of the Department of Medicine at the University of Maryland, however, Dr. Theodore E. Woodward, was an infectious diseases specialist who possessed an interest in Rocky Mountain spotted fever, a subject about which he had published a great deal. Largely because of his mentorship, I left Baltimore with a profound interest in infectious diseases. When I moved to Boston in 1978 for my internship at Boston City Hospital, however, tick-borne diseases were not on the top of my mind.

During the next three years, two events occurred that would bring these diseases back into focus for me. First, articles began appearing in prominent medical journals about a new entity in the coastal Connecticut area. Patients were falling ill with various symptoms that seemed to be related to tick bites. Second, I had relatives who had just moved into the Lyme area. One of them was stricken with a bizarre arthritis that initially defied diagnosis. The children developed rashes on more than one occasion following tick bites. Gradually, these two events merged into one—Lyme disease. Since it appeared to be a novel infection that affected people whom I knew personally, I began to follow this "new disease" with more than just a passing interest.

Although my career path shifted from infectious diseases to emergency medicine, my interest in Lyme disease stuck. This was about the time that I became infected myself—with the writing bug. I began to write both fiction and nonfiction. My first query letter to *Boston Magazine* suggested writing a medical detective story about the history of Lyme disease. The editor rejected my proposal, but what resulted was a series of other stories, each of which centered on medical epidemiology. But the idea expressed in that original query letter never disappeared from my mind.

Over the years, the notion of writing a book on the subject resurfaced, and as a practicing physician, I became interested in the medical aspects of the disease. In my emergency department practice, I would occasionally encounter patients with odd rashes, swollen joints, unexplained fevers, peculiar neurological symptoms, or precipitous cardiac arrhythmias that were caused by Lyme disease. Even as early as the early 1990s, I began to resurrect the idea of writing about the history of Lyme disease—this time in a book-length format. My first discussion (for another magazine article) with Polly Murray was in 1988; however, the first interviews that were specific for this book date back to 1993—a full ten years before publication. After I completed some of the initial research, administrative responsibilities pulled me away from writing for a number of years.

Interestingly, when I tried to reinterview some of these same individuals in 2001 and 2002, many of them, who had previously been quite generous with their time, were now "unavailable" for interview. Some said that they were too busy, some simply elected not to speak with me, and still others just never returned phone messages or E-mails. Something had changed.

I believe the reason for their change of heart is a lack of comfort in going on record because of the increasing politicization of Lyme disease. The polarity has increased; the stakes have increased. The tactics of both sides have become increasingly aggressive and personalized.

This has limited my primary source material for later parts of the book. I have tried to fill in these gaps, when they existed, by using other sources—published works, public domain testimony, and "off-the-record" comments—and by trying to corroborate them with other secondary sources. When there have been differences of opinion, I have tried to express those differences as clearly as possible. Undoubtedly, some people from both sides of this divide will feel that I have misstated their positions. If so, perhaps this will be a mark of success.

As regards sources, although I have interviewed many dozens of people over the years, there are certainly people who have played a role in this story with whom I have not spoken. I have tried to be as inclusive as possible, in terms of both numbers of individuals contacted and the perspectives from which they view the issues. With a story this big, however, it was impossible to speak directly with everyone involved. To those whom I have left out, I apologize.

Fortunately for the plot, this somewhat protracted gestational period was advantageous. Many of the story lines were in embryonic, or at best, juvenile stages a decade ago, but have now reached maturity, though perhaps not old age. The ten-year gestational period has allowed me to include twists and turns in the story that add to its interest. This same statement might be true if I were to wait another ten years, but there is value in putting pen to paper, even if the entire story has not yet played out. In another ten years, some of the principal players may no longer be alive. Memories will be that much foggier, and trails will be that much colder.

More important, this is not simply a book about Lyme disease, but a tale about scientific inquiry, as it exists in a cultural context. All of the individuals with whom I spoke struck me as being honest people who believed in their positions. The polarity of the Lyme communities is one of the best contemporary examples I can imagine of Thomas Kuhn's paradigm hypothesis of scientific growth. Some believe we are in the midst of a paradigm shift. If we are, I do not pretend to know when this shift will occur or how it will be resolved.

At the same time, the reader must realize that the story of Lyme disease, like most if not all stories about the biological sciences, is still evolving. Precisely where it will end cannot be predicted at the present time, although we know so much more now than we did ten years ago when I first began this project. The one thing about which I am certain is that the story up until now is one worth writing.

ACKNOWLEDGMENTS

I doubt that authors truly understand what they are getting themselves into when deciding to write a first book. Early passion for an idea rapidly becomes bogged down by emotional and logistical impediments. Both fiction and nonfiction have their own idiosyncratic hurtles, and I certainly did not anticipate many of those that this project offered. Many people helped me to overcome these obstacles.

One person who laid the seed for my interest in this subject ironically predated the term "Lyme disease." Dr. Theodore Woodward, my mentor in medical school, whose interest in tick-borne diseases in general and Rocky Mountain spotted fever in particular, is partially responsible for my current fascination with these diseases. Another is a person whom I have never met in person, Berton Roueche, whose books I began to reading as a teenager. His medical detective stories that appeared for decades in *The New Yorker* served as a model for my first foray into that genre—a series of articles that appeared in *Boston Magazine* and the *Ladies' Home Journal.*

The idea for a book-length medical detective story about Lyme disease flowed naturally from all of these sources. As regards this particular project, I would like to sincerely thank Amy Fleming, a good friend who served as first editor. Her careful reading ensured that the words did not come out too doctorly, too obtuse, or too awkward. Her effect on the language and flow of the book has been tremendous and her thoughtful and insightful comments clearly improved the final product. I would also like to thank Beth Lieber, who persevered and assisted me with the tremendous task of organizing the mountains of supporting documents without which this book could never have been published. Last, I would like to thank Jessie Dolch for her expert and obsessive copyediting.

I would also like to thank all of the people who took the time from their busy schedules to help me get the story right. I apologize in advance for those I have inadvertently left off of this important list. Drs. David Snydman, Stephen Malawista, Sam Donta, Ed Masters, Brian Fallon, John Anderson, Klaus Weber, and Rudolph Ackermann all helped me to fill in various aspects of the story line. Polly Murray also stands out as someone who went above and beyond to help me acquire facts and understand events some of which occurred more than twenty-five years ago; she deserves special recognition. I should also like to specifically thank Dr. Willy Burgdorfer, for his encouragement, his generosity with his time, and his advice over the years.

Last I would like to thank the staff at Yale University Press, especially Jean Thomson Black, whose faith in the original concept, and patience with me as I negotiated the obstacles and completed the book, never faltered.

For all of this help, any story such as this depends on both individual recollections and perspective. I have tried my best to get at the "truth," but approximating the truth in such situations is not always a simple matter. I have tried to communicate honestly those differences of opinion that exist.

Following the lead of Klaus Weber and Hans-Walter Pfister, I have divided the chronology of Lyme disease into three natural segments; however, I have altered the break point between their second and third segments to better account for some of the findings in the United States. The first period is the time between the first description of acrodermatitis chronica atrophicans in 1883 and the time when penicillin was first used to treat the disease in 1945. The second segment begins with that finding and ends just before the outbreak of "childhood arthritis" in Lyme, Connecticut. The last segment is from 1975 until the discovery of the causative agent of Lyme disease.

1883 to 1945

1883: The German physician Alfred Buchwald first describes acrodermatitis chronica atrophicans (ACA), the most chronic skin form of what is now known to be part of Lyme disease.

1902: Karl Herxheimer and Kuno Hartmann describe more cases of ACA and give the entity its name.

1909: Arvid Afzelius first describes erythema migrans (EM) at an oral presentation in Stockholm, Sweden (published in 1910). He linked his case to a tick bite.

1910: Wilhelm Balban describes three additional cases of EM in Austria.

1911: Swiss physician Jean Louis Burckhardt first describes what is now called lymphocytoma, the third skin manifestation of Lyme disease.

1913: Benjamin Lipschutz describes more cases of EM but uses the term erythema chronicum migrans (ECM).

1921: Afzelius expands his case series to six patients.

1922: Dr. Charles Garin and Dr. Bujadoux describe a patient with a large rash (EM) and a neurological disease (that would later be related to Lyme disease and be called Bannwarth's syndrome). They reported their findings in an obscure French medical journal.

1923: Lipschutz describes a patient with ECM with two lesions.

1929: Mulzer and Keining coin the term *lymphocytoma*.

1930: Sven Hellerstrom first connects ECM with meningitis.

1941: Alfred Bannwarth describes fifteen cases of chronic lymphocytic meningitis with severe pain from inflamed nerve roots. He does not make the connection with the EM rash, which at least one patient had, nor is he aware of the report by Garin and Bujadoux.

1943: Bo Bafverstedt, a Swede, describes more cases of lymphocytoma and begins to make links between these three forms of skin lesions (EM, ACA, and lymphocytoma).

1946 to 1974

1948: Carl Lennhoff reports seeing spirochetes in biopsy specimens of EM (as well as many other skin diseases).

1949: Nils Thyresson, from Stockholm, treats patients with ACA with penicillin, with moderate success.

1949: Georges Schaltenbrand reports eight cases of Bannwarth's syndrome, one of whom has arthritis.

1950: Hellerstrom publishes another case of meningitis and EM successfully treated with penicillin.

1950: G. E. Bianchi shows that penicillin helps patients with lymphocytoma.

1954: Jean-Marie Paschoud in Switzerland shows a relation between tick bite, lymphocytoma, EM, and Bannwarth's syndrome. He performs successful skin biopsy transmission experiments with lymphocytoma.

1954: Hans Gotz performs transmission experiments showing that skin biopsy from patients with ACA will produce the disease if transplanted into a second person's skin.

1955: Erich Binder and colleagues reproduce Gotz's skin transplant transmission experiments with EM.

1962: Schaltenbrand reports on more cases of painful radiculoneuritis and relates this to tick bites and EM.

1966: Hanns Christian Hopf demonstrates neurological involvement in patients with ACA. One of his patients has arthritis.

1970: Rudolph Scrimenti reports the first domestically acquired case of EM in the United States. Aware of the European literature, he successfully treats it with penicillin.

1970: The first case of babesiosis in a patient with an intact spleen is reported. The patient was infected on Nantucket Island. Andrew Spielman begins to investigate the ticks on the island.

1971: Richard Kelly, a pathologist working in Tennessee, discovers an artificial medium on which to grow the borrelia that causes relapsing fever.

1973: Peter Horstrup and Rudolph Ackermann further extend the findings on Bannwarth's syndrome and "resurrect" the lost article of Garin and Bujadoux.

1974: Klaus Weber reports on a patient with EM and meningitis who is cured by penicillin. He postulates a bacterial origin, specifically a borrelial or rickettsial agent or *Francisella tularensis* (the agent of tularemia).

Mid-1970s: Jorge Benach (from Stonybrook, New York) and John Anderson and Lou Magnarelli (from the Connecticut Agricultural Experiment Station) all begin to work on the upsurge in tick-borne diseases in the Northeast. Both groups study Rocky Mountain spotted fever, and both collaborate with Willy Burgdorfer at the Rocky Mountain Laboratories.

1975 to 1983

1975 (early October): Polly Murray calls the Connecticut authorities, questioning whether a new disease is plaguing her family and neighbors.

1975 (late October): Judith Mensch calls the same state authorities shortly after Mrs. Murray's call. She also calls Allen Steere at Yale University School of Medicine.

1975 (late October): David Snydman begins to investigate the concerns of Mrs. Murray and Mrs. Mensch.

1975 (November): Polly Murray has her first appointment at the Yale University Rheumatology Clinic. The Yale group and Snydman commit to their investigation.

1976: William Mast and William Burrows, two doctors at the U.S. Navy Submarine Medical Center in Groton, Connecticut, describe four cases of EM in *JAMA*; they update this report in a later letter to the editor to ten cases.

1976: The Yale group, now prepared to study the new disease "in season," connects the cardiac, neurological, and skin manifestations of the new disease, pulling together information that had been present in Europe but never included in a large epidemiological study. Given these new findings, the term *Lyme arthritis* is changed to *Lyme disease.*

1976: Joe Dowhan, a biologist with the Department of Environmental Protection for the State of Connecticut, is the first person to bring in the tick that caused his EM rash, later identified as the *Ixodes scapularis* (or deer) tick.

1977: Steere, Snydman, Stephen Malawista, and others describe a new form of arthritis called Lyme arthritis. They launch a several-pronged investigation that soon makes the connection with ticks and better describes the full picture of the disease.

1977: Edgar Grunwaldt of Shelter Island reports on another case of babesiosis. He has also been seeing EM for several years.

1978: Andrew Spielman declares that *Ixodes dammini* is a new and distinct tick species in the northeastern United States and is the vector for both Lyme disease and babesiosis in those areas. (In 1993, this finding was reversed by research directed by James Oliver, and the name reverted back to *I. scapularis.*)

1980: The Yale group proves definitively that antibiotics are effective for treating EM and decreasing later manifestations of Lyme disease.

1981: Weber postulates that the persistence of live organism in the body is responsible for later manifestations of the disease and recommends treatment with antibiotics.

1982: Burgdorfer, Barbour, Benach, and colleagues publish their work on discovering the long-sought organism, later named *Borrelia burgdorferi.*

1983: The First International Symposium on Lyme Disease is held in New Haven, Connecticut.

1983 and 1984: Several Europeans find that the same organism, *B. burgdorferi,* is causing lymphocytoma, ACA, and EM in Europe.

1 • A Family Under Siege

For the Murray family of Lyme, Connecticut, things came to a head during the summer and fall of 1975.

Polly and Gil Murray and their four children lived on Joshuatown Road, a picture-postcard country road that Senator Ted Kennedy once called one of the prettiest in New England. Roughly paralleling the nearby Connecticut River, the rural road cuts through lush forest as it stretches from Whalebone Creek to Hamburg Cove. Low fieldstone walls randomly crisscross the woodland, marking ancient boundaries. The route to the Murray house from the main road meanders over hills that gently rise and fall and then rise again to another breathtaking view. When the forest is thick with leaves and growth, one can barely see the homes from the road.

By the mid-1970s, the Murrays had lived in this idyllic spot for more than fifteen years. And for most of that time, Mrs. Murray (Figure 1), an artist with a soft voice and gentle manner, began experiencing a baffling array of physical symptoms that eluded diagnosis by doctor after doctor. She suffered from odd rashes, unexplained neurological symptoms, and painful, swollen joints. All these symptoms got progressively worse during the late 1960s and early 1970s. The arthri-

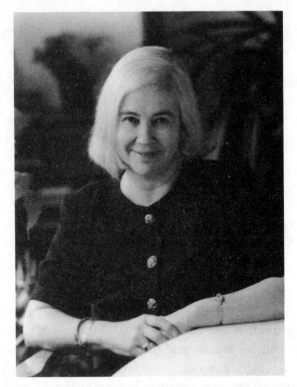

Figure 1. Polly Murray's persistence to determine what was plaguing her and her family's health eventually led to the discovery of Lyme disease. (Courtesy of Scandinavian Photography, Erik K. Johnson.)

tis at times prevented her from painting. In 1971 alone, she was hospitalized three times.

Doctor after doctor meted out diagnosis after diagnosis, each one fitting some of the symptoms, but not others. Physicians in two states tested Mrs. Murray for every possible condition. When she didn't get satisfactory answers from her doctors, she set about researching the matter on her own in the medical library at the Yale University School of Medicine. There, she spent hours poring over volumes of thick medical textbooks. One of the diseases, systemic lupus erythematosus (lupus), seemed to fit some of her symptoms, but blood tests were negative.

As her medical record grew thicker and thicker, doctors began to suspect that hypochondria was behind the aches and pains that came and went seemingly at will. Some of Mrs. Murray's relatives who were not nearby to witness her health problems thought that all she needed was a restful vacation. At some of her lowest points, she described feeling alone, defeated, and misunderstood. But she never doubted the reality of her symptoms.

When a doctor sees a patient for any complaint, he has to come up with a diagnosis, or a cause for the patient's symptoms. Armed with the correct cause, the physician can initiate the proper therapy. Doctors call this exercise *differential diagnosis*—a lofty term for what could as easily be called problem solving or even puzzle solving. The patient gives the doctor pieces of a puzzle, and the doctor puts them together in a way that makes sense. A puzzle with few pieces is easier to put together than one with many pieces; one that has a defined outline or whose picture is shown on the box is easier than one whose outcome is unknown. A puzzle whose pieces are sharp and distinct is easier to solve than one whose pieces are fuzzy or ambiguous.

The physician begins by trying to find as many pieces to the puzzle as he can. A good doctor asks lots of questions and listens carefully to the answers to obtain the clearest and least ambiguous pieces. He pokes and prods when performing the physical examination to uncover additional clues. Armed with these bits of information, he forms a hypothesis about what illness troubles the patient.

At times, all of the pieces fit neatly together and a diagnosis is clear. At others times, even after the physician has obtained all of the relevant information, the diagnosis may still remain elusive because all of the pieces to the puzzle might not be in the box. Other pieces may be red herrings, or extra pieces that don't belong to a particular puzzle. Part of what distinguishes an excellent diagnostician from a less accomplished one is the ability to figure out which pieces belong to which puzzle.

A physician may be confident of his *working diagnosis*, as it is called, and decide to treat for that condition. This is called a *therapeutic trial*. If the patient improves, the diagnosis tends to be confirmed (although it does not prove the diagnosis because the patient may have gotten better without any treatment). Other times, the doctor may order laboratory tests or X rays to try to confirm or refute the initial hypothesis. The puzzle may be so unclear that the physician needs a few more pieces to be confident of the solution.

Take the example of a sore throat. Many conditions can cause a sore throat—some common, others unusual. It could simply be a viral or a bacterial infection. It might be an inflamed thyroid gland or perhaps a fish bone stuck in the throat. The doctor starts with a careful history to elicit information that will help him rank the possible diagnoses in order of likelihood. How long have the symptoms lasted? Has the patient been exposed to anyone with strep throat or mononucleosis? Has the patient had a fever? Does the patient have any history of thyroid problems?

The doctor then uses the physical examination to narrow the list of possibilities. An enlarged, tender thyroid gland suggests thyroiditis. Pus in the throat with fever suggests an infection—maybe mononucleosis, perhaps strep throat, or possibly thrush. Red spots on the roof of the mouth and swollen glands in the back of the neck make mono more likely, especially in a young person. Say the patient has had two days of sore throat, a fever of 102 degrees, and pus on the tonsils. The doctor may decide that the likeliest problem is strep throat (this is the working diagnosis) and prescribe antibiotics without further testing (a therapeutic trial). Or he may choose to get a throat culture or a blood test for mono to further increase the confidence in his diagnosis and then treat accordingly.

Polly Murray's doctors performed this exercise of differential diagnosis each time they saw her. The problem was that her symptoms simply didn't fit the pattern of any of the diseases with which they were familiar. She had some symptoms of one disease, other symptoms of another. Abnormal physical findings came and went. Lab tests and X rays couldn't pinpoint a specific diagnosis. Her illness simply was not consistent with what was written in the textbooks.

And if that wasn't bad enough, in the mid-1970s, the rest of her family began getting sick, too. In November 1974, her oldest son,

Sandy, developed a rash and painful joints. Around Christmas, came a swollen and droopy left eyelid, ear pain, and severe pain and stiffness throughout his body, mostly on the left side. It even hurt for him to open his jaw. At that time, Mrs. Murray heard of a man in Lyme with a history of an expanding red rash who had what was first thought to be a stroke because of facial drooping. In the hospital, he was diagnosed with viral meningitis, although in retrospect, he probably had Bell's palsy.

Most cases of Bell's palsy are said to be *idiopathic*—that is, doctors don't know what causes it. What is known is that the facial nerve, which controls the muscles that make the human face so expressive, snakes its way through a narrow, bony canal as it exits the skull. There's no room to spare. So inflammation (which is thought to be due to viral infection) causes the nerve to swell, the resultant pressure chokes the nerve, and the facial muscles stop working, a condition that can be either temporary or permanent. More recent research has suggested that Bell's palsy is often caused by infection by a herpesvirus. Other causes of facial nerve paralysis include diseases such as sarcoidosis, multiple sclerosis, and Guillain-Barré syndrome or, of course, trauma to the nerve from a fracture.

In January of 1975, Gil Murray developed pain in his left knee, thought to be arthritis or tendinitis. But it didn't stop there. "In the early summer," recalls Mrs. Murray, "my youngest son, Todd, had an expanding red rash behind one of his knees, developed a severe headache and flulike illness, and then had multiple ringlike rashes all over his body." Later in the summer, Todd and Sandy were both on crutches because of severely swollen knees. Mr. Murray also had an odd red rash, and the Murrays' daughter, Wendy, had a bad sore throat. Todd, eleven years old that summer, remembers: "From the point of a view of a kid, it was also upsetting because I had been very athletic; it was pretty jarring to suddenly be using crutches off and on for months at a time and not [be] able to interact with my peers the way I had. It was scary in terms of having a disease that nobody knew how to fix. And as the symptoms progressed, there was a feeling of 'what will be next? What will be the next problem?'"

At one low point, the entire family was sick; even the family dogs suffered from rashes and lameness. Mrs. Murray estimates that from the beginning of their medical problems to their final diagnosis, she and her family consulted about thirty physicians.

The frustration was incredible; as Mrs. Murray wrote in a letter to the editor of the *New England Journal of Medicine:* "Some of the doctors whom I saw were supportive and open to the possibility of the unknown; however, they and medical science could not figure out what our trouble was. On the other hand, many of the physicians I encountered tended to fit me into the category of a hypochondriac. It was suggested that I was obsessed, bored, and depressed and that I was bothering busy doctors; some later suggested that the entire family had a psychogenic problem. I will admit that my behavior became insistent and constantly questioning."

Mrs. Murray's frustration was also fueled by the fact that she became aware of other cases of mystery symptoms in her community. Networking with other parents, she began compiling a list of people who had symptoms remarkably similar to those her own family was suffering. She was convinced that some unknown, maybe new, disease was affecting her family and her neighbors.

Among the doctors Polly Murray eventually consulted was a Harvard rheumatologist-immunologist named Dr. Peter Schur who had been supportive and believed that, although he couldn't satisfactorily explain or diagnose the condition, something real was going on. He understood her frustration, but logistically, it would have been difficult for a doctor in one state to pursue a major epidemiological undertaking in another state. "She saw me for another opinion," Dr. Schur says. "I remember she was very convincing in describing this cluster of kids with juvenile rheumatoid arthritis [JRA] in her community. I said that would be very intriguing because we're always looking for clusters of patients with JRA or lupus and these diseases [to try to find their cause]. I suggested she pursue it by contacting the CDC [Centers for Disease Control and Prevention] or the Connecticut health department."

Mrs. Murray sent Dr. Schur a follow-up letter on October 6, 1975, detailing the sequence of events. Partly at his suggestion, she called the Connecticut State Health Department on Thursday, October 16.

She recounted to the person on the phone the family saga, as well as the fact that she knew of other families that had been similarly affected. She also said that there were at least four children in the East Haddam elementary school with persistent joint problems and that some of them lived on the same street. She wondered aloud why, if JRA was such a rare disease, so much of it could be found in the local area.

The response was simultaneously polite and noncommittal. Essentially, Mrs. Murray was told, arthritis is not a communicable disease; there's nothing we can do for you.

She had lived with this phenomenon for years and had begun to recognize its pattern—whatever the "it" was. First, a red rash would begin and spread to enormous proportions. Sometimes, the rash would look like a bull's-eye, with concentric red rings spreading out from a center. The rash was usually followed by neurological symptoms and swollen joints. All the symptoms would wax and wane. Sometimes, she would schedule an appointment with a specialist, and by the time the appointment would roll around, the symptom would have vanished. One can imagine what this does for a patient's credibility. But that was part of the pattern; symptoms would come and go for no apparent reason.

Some of the local physicians whom the Murrays consulted were interested and supportive; others acted as if they were threatened by their inability to solve the puzzle. One, whom Mrs. Murray calls Dr. Esbensen in her book *The Widening Circle*, referred to the family's symptoms as "annoying" and even said, "Oh no, not again," when another family member appeared with new symptoms. Polly Murray took her son Todd to see this doctor on the same October day that she telephoned the state health department. When Mrs. Murray told him of the call, she says, "He was incensed [and said] 'by whose authority did you do that? What are you doing, stirring up trouble?'" With that, he essentially dismissed them from his practice, telling Mrs. Murray that he wanted them to find another rheumatologist by their next appointment (which happened to be only five days later).

Todd, now a physician himself, still has a vivid memory of that interaction from the perspective of a young boy: "I remember that visit very clearly. The doctor had a bedside manner that was pretty abrupt. He didn't seem to respond well to my mom's questions about a possible connection between my illness, and my brother's and father's illnesses, despite the fact that he had seen both of them, too. Then I remember him doing the arthrocentesis on me." Arthrocentesis is a procedure whereby fluid is taken from a joint for analysis. The doctor paints the skin with iodine, numbs the area with local anesthetic, and then inserts a needle attached to a syringe. Once the needle is inside the joint space, the doctor aspirates the fluid. Mother and son had to silently endure this final insult after the man had already verbally assaulted them.

"Afterwards, as I recall, he basically kicked her out of his office," says Todd, "sort of 'don't come back.' He was pretty rude. He handed her the samples [of fluid] to drive over to the lab. And I remember my mom was in tears as we drove over."

Fortunately, both for the Murrays and for the medical profession, other physicians were far more supportive. One of those was a local doctor named David Nelligan. "He suggested going down to Yale to see what they could find out, and he helped arrange an appointment for me in their rheumatology clinic with a Dr. Robert Gifford," Mrs. Murray recalls. The date of the appointment was November 20, 1975.

2 • A Little Girl's Knee

Kids are forever coming down with one thing or another; it's part of growing up. So when fourth-grader Anne Mensch came home from school one day in late October 1975 complaining that her knee hurt, her mother Judith Mensch wasn't particularly concerned. She and her husband, Arthur, a pathologist at a hospital not far from their home on the Connecticut shore, looked at Anne's knee and found it mildly swollen and a little warm to the touch, but nothing alarming. "I basically ignored it," Mrs. Mensch remembers, "and we sent her back to school the next day."

The next morning, however, the school nurse called and told Mrs. Mensch that Anne was in quite a bit of pain. "I called my husband and we took Anne to see an orthopedist in New London," recalls Mrs. Mensch. "I don't know why, because we had a pediatrician in Essex, but we went up to see the orthopedist. After examining her knee and finding it swollen with fluid, the orthopedist made a presumptive diagnosis of osteomyelitis and decided to hospitalize Anne at Lawrence and Memorial Hospital in New London." Osteomyelitis, as Dr. Mensch knew, is a serious bone infection that can sometimes spread to an adjacent joint. Finding out the particular cause of the infection—what specific species of bacteria—is important in de-

termining the best antibiotic therapy; therefore, the consulting orthopedist performed an arthrocentesis and drained the amber-colored
fluid from the joint. He then started Anne on a course of intravenous
antibiotics, the usual treatment for osteomyelitis. "The next morning," says Anne's mother, "her other knee began to swell; at this point
she was basically unable to move her legs because of pain. She was
hospitalized for four or five days receiving intravenous antibiotics."

After the orthopedist aspirated the joint fluid from Anne's knee,
he sent some of it to the hospital's microbiology lab to see whether
bacteria could be grown in culture. For this test, a small amount of
the fluid is placed on a special plate containing nutrients that bacteria
need to grow. The plate is then incubated at a temperature that is
conducive to the growth of bacteria. If bacteria grow, the microbiology technicians can examine the microorganism to determine precisely what strain it is and which antibiotics will kill it.

If the culture were positive, it would confirm the doctor's diagnosis of a bacterial osteomyelitis involving the joint and would furthermore guide the doctor's treatment. But the culture proved negative for bacteria. Dr. Mensch, who was also on staff at the hospital,
ran special tests to look for viruses and other microorganisms, but
those tests were equally unrevealing.

"So the orthopedist discontinued the antibiotics," remembers
Mrs. Mensch, "and decided that Anne had juvenile rheumatoid arthritis. I was very upset. Anne came home from the hospital in a
wheelchair. She was taking ten adult aspirin every day and she cried
constantly."

A petite girl with light brown hair and a fair complexion, Anne
weighed only forty pounds. When Mrs. Mensch looked at her little
girl sick in a wheelchair, she foresaw a child with a chronic disability.
"She had been a perfectly normal eight-year-old one day, and now
she was depressed. Once she was able to walk again, I'd find her sitting
at the bottom of the stairs crying. She went back to school, still on the
aspirin. At times, I would find her crying for no reason whatsoever. I
called her doctor to ask if aspirin could cause depression and I was
told 'no.' He thought that probably taking the aspirin just made her

feel sick. Finally I stopped the aspirin myself and she seemed to bounce back to normal."

And she has remained that way ever since.

Another story might have ended here, but not this one—partly because Judith Mensch just isn't the kind of person willing to accept a diagnosis of a chronic, incurable, and potentially debilitating disease. She was motivated by the same feelings, among which is denial, that any other parent experiences when his or her child is diagnosed with such an illness.

But there was something else that just didn't sit right with Judith Mensch. In 1968, the Mensches arrived in their new home situated on a two-acre lot in Old Lyme, Connecticut, a sleepy hamlet located roughly halfway between New York and Boston on the shore of Long Island Sound. Back then, it was a quiet, rural area with a couple of lakes and lots of forest. There was the marina on the Connecticut River and a few stores in town—one drugstore, one supermarket, a library, and a few specialty shops. By 1975, about four thousand people lived there. There were far more trees in the area than people.

"I grew up in New York City; I knew everybody in my building and that was it," says Mrs. Mensch. "But in Old Lyme, I knew everyone and they knew me, by face if not by name. In the supermarket, people would stop me and ask how Anne was. And they would mention 'oh by the way, do you know that so-and-so's son or daughter also has juvenile rheumatoid arthritis?' " The more she thought about it, the more it seemed that something was dreadfully wrong. In fact, she didn't need to look any farther than the family next door to confirm her suspicions.

John and Greta Paterson and their two daughters lived next to the Mensches in 1975. Their youngest daughter, Aileen, had first been hospitalized with arthritis of the right knee in the winter of 1973 when she was nine years old. She, too, had fluid aspirated from her knee, fluid that in her case also failed to lead to a specific diagnosis. After about a week in the hospital, her doctors concluded that she had JRA and started her on aspirin therapy. The next winter, her other knee swelled, and in July of 1975, just three months before Anne Mensch's problem, Aileen Paterson was hospitalized a second time with her arthritis.

"I didn't like being there," Aileen remembers. "I didn't like the food, the nurses, or the treatments. They would put hot and cold packs on my knees to reduce the swelling. The cold packs hurt and the hot packs were too hot and neither of them helped. I remember doing jigsaw puzzles. And I remember my parents being really worried. . . . I was on aspirin and I felt depressed and embarrassed about being sick." Just as the Murray family's symptoms came and went for no apparent reason, Aileen remembers, "when I left the hospital, the swelling just went away on its own."

During that same time, her father, John Paterson, also developed arthritis.

But Judith Mensch had more than just the Patersons on her mind as she sought to explain her daughter's illness. "Another eleven-year-old on the street also had juvenile rheumatoid arthritis, as did the six-year-old girl around the corner," Mrs. Mensch says. "That second girl's mother also had arthritis. And my husband's partner's son, who lived in the general area, also had arthritis." In New York, Mrs. Mensch hadn't known anyone with arthritis; now, in a town whose entire population was that of several square blocks in Manhattan, she personally knew six people with it—four of them on her own street!

Arthritis is a generic term that means inflammation of joints. Because each kind of arthritis may be treated differently, establishing the exact kind is important. One clue is the pattern of joint involvement.

Sometimes only a single joint is affected. This is called *monoarticular* (one joint) arthritis and often results from an injury or infection that is localized to the affected joint. Gout is another fairly common cause of monoarticular arthritis. Other times, a patient's entire body can be wracked with painful swelling and inflammation from the fingers to the toes—*polyarticular* (many joints) arthritis. One kind of polyarticular arthritis is rheumatoid arthritis. Of rheumatoid arthritis, Sir William Osler, one of the fathers of modern medicine, wrote in 1892 in his famous medical text *The Principles and Practice of Medicine*, "There are cases in which pain of an agonizing character is an almost constant symptom, requiring for years the use of morphia."

In still other patients, only a few joints will be involved, such as a knee and an ankle or two knees and a wrist. This is called *oligoarticular* (a few joints) arthritis. One example of this is rheumatic fever, which can follow an untreated streptococcal infection.

The temporal sequence of joint involvement can also help doctors determine what kind of arthritis a patient has. Did both knees and the wrist become inflamed at the same time? Or did the left knee get better and then the wrist became sore? Doctors will look for other clues as well: the patient's age and sex; the presence or absence of fever or trauma; any associated disease in other organs, such as the skin, liver, heart, lungs, or eyes; even what medications the patient is taking.

Arthritis has dozens of causes, and a variety of clinical and laboratory clues can help distinguish among them. Some kinds of arthritis have specific, well-established causes that are relatively easy to diagnose. Gout is a good example. Patients with gout can have an acute arthritis, usually of the monoarticular variety, that results from uric acid crystals that accumulate in a joint (classically at the base of the large toe although it can happen anywhere in the body). These crystals draw white blood cells into the joint where they release destructive enzymes that cause the inflammation.

Septic arthritis, or an infected joint, is another kind of arthritis whose etiology is clear-cut. Bacteria invade the joint; white blood cells follow in pursuit, trying to kill the bacteria. But in doing so, they produce the classic signs of inflammation: heat, redness, pain, and swelling.

For many kinds of arthritis, however, the cause of the inflammation is not so clear. A large group of such diseases, sometimes called *connective tissue diseases* and including lupus, rheumatoid arthritis, ankylosing spondylitis, and polymyositis, can often only be distinguished using the clues mentioned above as well as various lab tests.

Aspirating fluid from an arthritic joint and testing it is often helpful in establishing the precise cause of arthritis. For example, under a microscope, the fluid from a gouty joint will show uric acid crystals; in septic arthritis, bacteria can often be seen, and the microorganism will usually grow in culture. But in many of the afflictions affecting the joints for which the cause is unknown, the diagnosis remains one of exclusion. Crystals cannot be seen; bacteria do not grow; and none of the tests that indicate a specific disease is positive. Although the clinical picture may be unclear, these diseases frequently can be diagnosed with a modicum of certainty by putting together all the information and seeing whether the pattern matches the known pattern of a particular illness.

Juvenile rheumatoid arthritis is one such disease. It is not particularly common and usually strikes children rather than adults. It also falls into the basket of maladies called connective tissue diseases that have no established etiology. Juvenile rheumatoid arthritis, which is probably a group of diseases, has several different patterns. The most common is an oligoarticular arthritis that is seen in more than one-third of children who are diagnosed with JRA. The children are usually very young, and 80 percent of them are girls. Thirty percent of them have coexistent problems with the eyes, and 90 percent have certain kinds of circulating antibodies called antinuclear antibodies. The next most common type of JRA, a polyarticular arthritis, is also seen overwhelmingly in girls, and the age of onset is more variable.

About 20 percent of patients with JRA have what is called a systemic variety. This is seen more commonly in boys and is marked by high intermittent fevers; a pale red rash that can occur anywhere on the body; swollen liver, spleen, and lymph glands; inflammation of the lining of the chest and abdominal cavities; and abnormalities in blood cell counts (a high white cell count and a low red cell count). In addition, there are two other patterns of JRA—for a total of five different types.

Judith Mensch wasn't thinking about all of this when she began making phone calls; she just knew something wasn't right. She started talking to people. The more she talked, the more she became convinced that something was clearly wrong. She turned to local physicians.

"First, I called Anne's pediatrician, who was in Essex, and the man who covered for him, who was in Saybrook," she says. "I asked them how much JRA they saw. They both said they saw it but didn't know exactly how much. Records weren't computerized back then; there were no cross-records. So I then spoke to the two local general practitioners in town; I had seen each of them professionally for one thing or another over the years. Both were gracious with their time. They told me they did see JRA but didn't know how many cases they saw. And they said that most people from town saw doctors outside the town.

"Then I asked our orthopedist. He said I was overreacting and basically that I was 'a crazy Jewish mother' and that I should just let it go and that there was nothing we could do about it. I talked to people at the hospital, too; my husband was a doctor there so people would talk to me."

Peoples' reactions, though generally polite, were, at best, 'we see it but we don't know how much,' and at worst, dismissive. In an article she wrote years later in 1985, Mrs. Mensch recalled, "I cannot convey effectively the terrible frustration I felt. The physicians were receptive to my calls; certainly they would be, my husband was the only pathologist in the area, and they all knew of him. Everybody heard me, but nobody listened."

But Mrs. Mensch is not one to concede defeat easily, and like Mrs. Murray, she persisted: "Next I called the Connecticut State Health Department in Hartford. They didn't hang up on me but came very close to it; they had nothing to say except that JRA was not a contagious disease and they couldn't do anything about it." In fact, they were quite rude, she recalls.

Undaunted, Mrs. Mensch then called the Centers for Disease Control and Prevention (CDC, formerly called the Communicable

Disease Center) in Atlanta. The first person she spoke to "just listened to me rant and rave because at this point I was already ranting and raving and using language I'd rather forget."

Then she was subjected to a long sequence of "I'll transfer your call," and "Hold please," until she was finally transferred to a physician who took a few moments to speak with her. She recalls, "I don't know whether he was an epidemiologist or a psychiatrist, but he did calm me down." By sheer coincidence the man at the other end of the line knew of a doctor named Allen Steere, who had just begun his training in rheumatology at Yale University in New Haven, Connecticut. Dr. Steere had been at the CDC as an Epidemiology Intelligence Service (EIS) officer before his fellowship at Yale. Perhaps he could help. "So I called him," says Mrs. Mensch.

Polly Murray and Judith Mensch lived within a few miles of one another in adjacent towns. They both turned to Yale University School of Medicine for help. But they didn't know each other, and throughout this initial process and for many years afterward, they never met or spoke.

3 • The Broad Street Pump

History is sometimes made under the glare of spotlights, a crush of reporters, and the intense scrutiny of video cameras. On other occasions, a quiet series of seemingly routine events emerges as historically significant only with the passage of time and the perspective it provides.

October 1975, in New England, included examples of both.

The 1975 World Series between the Cincinnati Reds and the Boston Red Sox stretched on to seven games. Game six, which was delayed three days by incessant rain and finally ended with a twelfth-inning home run by Carlton Fisk, is still considered one of the finest games in series history. One fan recalls trying to follow the series at odd hours of the morning while traveling with his wife in Europe. But even with the three-day weather delay of game six, he still missed the entire series. He returned from abroad after the seventh and deciding game, which Cincinnati won, on October 22. The fan was David Snydman (Figure 2), then a twenty-nine-year-old physician. In his second year as an EIS officer with the CDC, Dr. Snydman was "on loan" to the State of Connecticut Department of Public Health, where he served as acting director of preventable diseases.

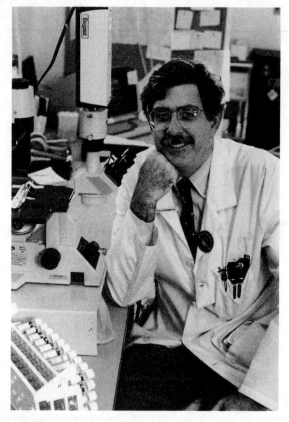

Figure 2. David Snydman, M.D., worked at the State of Connecticut Department of Health in 1975 when he began investigating an unusual outbreak of arthritis in the area around Lyme, Connecticut. (Courtesy of David Snydman, M.D.)

This CDC program, designed to train field epidemiologists, began in 1951, when twenty-one Public Health Service physicians were recruited to Atlanta to begin a two-year training period. The name "Epidemiology Intelligence Service" may have been designed to take advantage of the times: a Congress that was dealing with the Cold War and Korean conflict may have been more disposed toward funding an "intelligence service" rather than a mere epidemiology-training program.

The CDC's EIS officers are young doctors who serve for two to three years with the organization acquiring the experience of an epidemiologist and usually doing field work. The latter includes investigating real outbreaks of disease whose cause is unclear. EIS officers have played roles in eliminating smallpox and finding the causes of Legionnaire's disease and toxic shock syndrome, as well as many other outbreaks of disease, including AIDS. During the 1990s, however, their focus increasingly shifted toward other modern "plagues," such as obesity, tobacco use, and domestic violence.

Local health departments contact the CDC and request help on cases that are either unusually baffling or that overwhelm the logistical support available in that particular local jurisdiction. The first director of the EIS, Alexander Langmuir, ordered his officers to keep their suitcases literally packed so that he could advertise the rapid response from the receipt of a telephone call seeking assistance to the arrival of that assistance. Since 1951, approximately twenty-five hundred EIS officers have graduated from the program. Allen Steere, of the Rheumatology Division at Yale University, was one. David Snydman was another.

When Dr. Snydman returned to the office after his European vacation, he found two handwritten messages waiting for him on his desk, both from women who reported what appeared to be an outbreak of arthritis in the area around Lyme, Connecticut. Snydman did not respond with the kind of bureaucratic brush-off that both women had been enduring time and time again. Having spent the prior year with the hepatitis division at the CDC, he was trained to investigate outbreaks of disease. Rather than being put off by information that didn't seem to make sense, he was intrigued. He wanted to see whether he could make any sense of the mystery.

The callers were Mrs. Polly Murray and Mrs. Judith Mensch. Dr. Snydman called them back and spoke to each of them. The women chronicled their stories and then gave him the names and numbers of other neighbors who were having similar problems. He phoned these people, too. After a short time, Snydman recalls thinking, "there's a heck of a lot of arthritis around here." That's when he decided to start investigating. As an epidemiologist, his work was to link the patients in time and space and by common circumstance.

According to Webster's dictionary, epidemiology is the science that investigates the causes and controls of epidemic disease, or disease that is prevalent in a given location, or one that is spreading rapidly. An epidemiologist is, of course, someone who studies or otherwise engages in the field of epidemiology. These definitions include two important elements. The first is that of control. Epidemiology is not simply an armchair exercise of counting numbers of cases of a given disease and plotting them into an insignificant graph to be filed for posterity. It is a science aimed at defining causality and, ultimately, at controlling the condition in question. Second, there is a major distinction between the general practitioner of medicine and the epidemiologist. The data acquired from the vantage point of an epidemiologist is very different from that of a physician, who may see only an individual case or just a few cases of the disease in question.

The individual physician focuses on caring for ill patients. While any physician plays epidemiologist to some extent, the epidemiologist directs his or her attention to *groups* of patients—a classic example of focusing on the forest versus the trees. The individual physician takes care of the individual trees; the epidemiologist examines the forest as a whole. From this vantage point, patterns emerge, sometimes providing clues to unsolved mysteries.

One of the most celebrated epidemiological investigations in the history of the science is one conducted by Dr. John Snow, an English anesthesiologist. In August and September of 1854, an outbreak of cholera roared through an area of London. Snow's account of the calamity is compelling: "The most terrible outbreak of cholera which ever occurred in this kingdom, is probably that which took place in Broad Street, Golden Square, and the adjoining streets, a few weeks ago. Within two hundred and fifty yards of the spot where Cambridge Street joins Broad Street, there were upwards of five hundred fatal attacks of cholera in ten days. The mortality in this limited area probably equals any that was ever caused in this country, even by the plague;

and it was much more sudden, as the greater number of cases terminated in a few hours."

Snow immediately sought the common link between the patients—in time, in space, and by common circumstance. Time and space were easy. The outbreak erupted on the evening and night of August 31. About 1 case of cholera per day was the baseline throughout late August in the immediate area. August 31 saw 56 cases and September 1 another 143! The next day 116 more people fell ill. Most, but not all, of the patients lived in the Golden Square area. Snow found a detailed street map (with a scale of thirty inches to the mile) of the area and began plotting cases, marking each cholera fatality on the map by drawing a small rectangular bar at the precise address of the victim.

A bit of background is crucial for understanding the significance of Snow's work. At the midpoint of the nineteenth century, another thirty years would pass before German physician Robert Koch discovered the cholera bacillus. Nevertheless, scientists of the mid-nineteenth century knew a number of things about the transmission of cholera. Of this state of knowledge at mid-century, epidemiologist H. Harold Scott wrote in 1934: "[C]holera spreads along the tracks of human intercourse, but never faster than people could travel, that is to say, it was transmitted by human agency. . . . If an island suffered, which had previously been free, the disease always appeared first in a seaport, introduced, of course, by some infected patient or his soiled belongings brought on the ship. Vice versa, it was noted that it never attacked crews of ships sailing from a cholera-free port and to an infected country until the vessel had entered the port and established contact."

Various theories surfaced in the prebacteriologic days of cholera. Some believed an "effluvia" theory, in which people became infected by simply approaching infected patients. According to John Lea's "geological" theory, cholera existed in the air but required certain chemical salts (only present in some geographical areas) to activate the poison. In Munich, Germany, Max Josef von Pettenkofer developed yet another theory. He maintained that four crucial factors—a factor X, individual susceptibility, soil conditions, and seasonal factors—led to the development of cholera and that all four needed to be present for the disease to occur.

In England, John Snow had established his theory on cholera years before the Golden Square outbreak. He maintained that cholera was spread by contact with infected particles from the evacuations of patients with cholera. He noted that in areas of overcrowding or where toilet facilities were absent or insufficient (such as in coal mines), cholera spread more rapidly. But large outbreaks were always waterborne, according to Snow. This was only a theory, however, and it competed with those of Lea and Pettenkofer. Thus, as August 1854 merged into September, Dr. Snow possessed the necessary tools and stood ready to test his hypothesis. London became his laboratory.

As Snow plotted the deaths on the London map, it was apparent that the majority of cases were tightly clustered around the Broad Street pump, which stood at the corner of Broad and Cambridge streets and supplied drinking water to the neighborhood. Ten cases, however, lived closer to another public water supply. When Snow interviewed these families, he learned that the majority had used the water from the Broad Street pump, either because they preferred it because of its supposed purity or because their duties took them by the intersection. For example, three children went to school near the pump and collected water on their way to classes. Others who did not live in the area acquired the disease by unknowingly taking the water that had been mixed into drinks at local pubs. Snow noted that one keeper of a coffee shop in the neighborhood told him on September 6 that she knew of nine customers who had died.

Snow also investigated other special cases that seemed to be exceptions to his theory. Some people who lived or worked in the area and who should have fallen ill did not. For example, at a workhouse on Poland Street (one block from the pump), only 5 of 535 inmates died of cholera, as opposed to an expected 100 or more if they had shared the same attack rate as that of their immediate neighbors. But Snow ascertained that the workhouse had its own well on the premises and did not use water from the tainted pump.

Equally noteworthy, of the more than seventy employees at a

brewery located even closer to the pump, none fell victim. In this case, the owner, a Mr. Huggins, supplied Snow with a unique story of how drinking on the job can save a life: "The men are allowed a certain quantity of malt liquor, and Mr. Huggins believes they do not drink water at all; and he is quite certain that the workmen never obtained water from the pump in the street."

Snow describes other special cases of people who either should have fallen ill but did not (healthy people who lived in the area) or who died of cholera but should not have (fatalities that occurred outside the Golden Square area). For example, he accounted for a case of cholera in an older woman that occurred in the Hampstead area, in the more fashionable West End, as follows: "I was informed by this lady's son that she had not been in the neighborhood of Broad Street for many months. A cart went from Broad Street to West End every day, and it was the custom to take out a large bottle of the water from the pump in Broad Street, as she preferred it. The water was taken on Thursday, August 31, and she drank of it in the evening, and also on Friday. She was seized with cholera on the evening of the latter day, and died on Saturday." The woman's niece, who visited the older woman in the West End, also drank some of the contaminated water and died.

Snow realized that some who drank the water did not fall ill and that others must have died outside the district, as many people fled the city in terror at the height of the outbreak. "The full extent of the calamity will probably never be known," Snow wrote. "The deficiencies I have mentioned, however, probably do not detract from the correctness of the map as a diagram of the topography of the outbreak." From this "topography," Snow concluded that the water from the pump was the direct cause of the outbreak.

Figure 3. As Snydman began his investigation in the Lyme area, he marked on a map where people afflicted with the mysterious symptoms lived, much as Dr. John Snow had done in the nineteenth century to help define and combat a deadly epidemic of cholera. (Courtesy of David Snydman, M.D.)

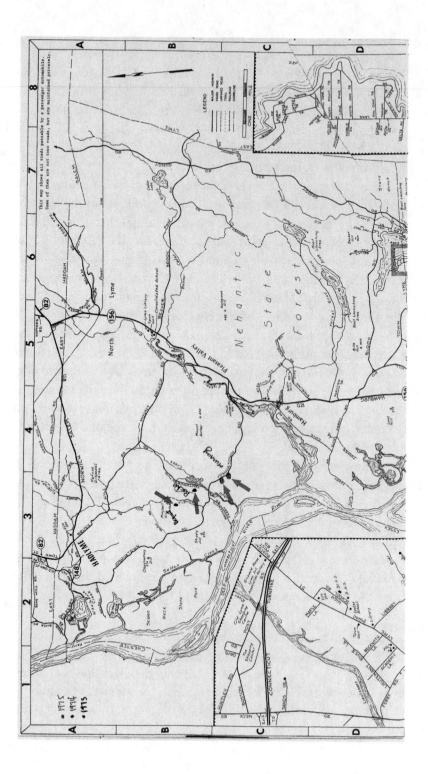

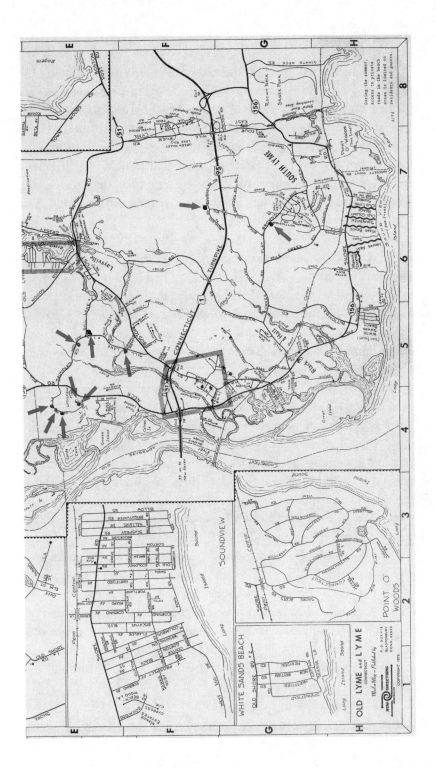

OLD LYME and LYME
CONNECTICUT
Made a Map—Published by
NEW DIRECTIONS   P.O. BOX 178
GLASTONBURY
CONN. 06033
COPYRIGHT 1975

On the basis of his convictions, Snow intervened: "I had an interview with the Board of Guardians of St. James' parish, on the evening of Thursday, September 7, and represented the above circumstances to them. In consequence of what I said, the handle of the pump was removed on the following day." New cases of cholera rapidly tapered off and the epidemic ended. Thus, looking at the phenomenon from the perspective of the forest, rather than merely the individual trees, or patients, Snow gathered information that led to the control of the epidemic.

While considerably less dramatic, Dr. David Snydman's job was essentially the same as Dr. Snow's. So, too, were his methods of attacking the problem. More than 120 years later, Snydman also set out with a map and a pencil. His initial goals were the same: to put these interesting stories into a context. The contextual elements that Snydman looked for were the same as Snow's—linking the patients in time, space, and circumstance.

The Connecticut epidemiologist's first round of phone calls quickly established that, indeed, "something" unusual was going on. There was, however, one factor that made Snydman's job substantially more difficult than Snow's. In the latter case, cholera was a well-known "something" to physicians of the era, and Snow had been interested in its transmission for some time. So although much about cholera was still unknown in the mid-nineteenth century, there was a definition and a form and a name—cholera—for the "something" that attracted Snow's attention.

At the outset, the "something" that Snydman was beginning to investigate had no definition, no form, and no name. This is a vitally important point. Snow knew what he was looking for; Snydman could not. But both men had one important thing in common: a method by which to accomplish their task—the scientific method of making observations (collecting data), crafting a hypothesis to explain the data, and then performing experiments to prove (or disprove) the validity of the hypothesis.

To begin collecting data, Snydman turned to two advantages that he did have over Snow: the telephone and the automobile. After he called Mrs. Murray, Mrs. Mensch, and the people to whom these women referred him, he began recording information—where they lived, how old they were, when their symptoms began, and what those symptoms were. He obtained a map of the area and then drove to their houses and carefully marked the locations on the map, using a different code for people affected in different years (Figure 3). Just as London had been Snow's laboratory, so Lyme became Snydman's.

And just as patterns began to emerge for Snow, so, too, they did for Snydman. Most of the affected people were children. Most were tightly clustered in the more rural areas of the towns. Most fell sick during the warmer months of the year. Snydman pursued several courses of action. First, following standard operating procedures of the CDC, he notified his superiors at the CDC that there seemed to be a cluster of arthritis that he planned to investigate. On December 1, 1975, Snydman sent his routine monthly progress report to his direct supervisor, Dr. J. Lyle Conrad, director of field services with the bureau of epidemiology at the CDC.

Under the heading "new investigations," he noted a cluster of hepatitis in Killingly and an unusual case of leprosy in Stamford. But the lead entry of that report is titled "Juvenile Rheumatoid Arthritis, Old Lyme." "An apparent cluster of cases of 'juvenile rheumatoid arthritis' has been brought to our attention by parents in Old Lyme," he wrote. "Approximately 10–15 cases consistent with this diagnosis have occurred over the past 3 years (there are <1000 children and adolescents in this area). The diagnosis is obviously one of exclusion but rheumatic fever has been ruled out in most instances. There is definite temporal clustering of cases in summer and fall and definite spacial clustering within the town." He then explained how he planned to approach the investigation.

Next, he arranged to examine some of these children at the local health department. And last, he made a phone call to someone he knew at Yale.

4 • An Appointment in New Haven

Like all science, medical knowledge advances in various ways. Sometimes, a newly developed instrument yields a new way of looking at the world. New observations may change the way we interpret the world. Frequently, new facts emerge by means of steady research, an arduous process that comes in two basic forms—bench research and clinical research. Bench research, also known as basic science, is the activity that occurs in the laboratory with the help of powerful microscopes, rows of test tubes and beakers, colorful chemical reagents, and sophisticated machines. Bench research normally is directed at answering a clinical question that one hopes is useful someday to patients. But the actual work is insulated from the clinical arena. In fact, it often takes place in buildings far from the hospital.

This contrasts with clinical, or bedside, research, in which the investigator works directly with patients, testing a new drug or diagnostic equipment. This research occurs in hospital wards or clinics. Patients give their informed consent and elect whether or not to participate. The benefits of this kind of research are more direct, more easily visible. If a new drug is shown to work better than an old one to cure a disease, the benefit is clear and often makes the evening news or causes a stock price to skyrocket.

Neither kind of research is better than the other, and often, top-notch research efforts travel in both directions, from bench to bedside or vice versa. The styles of these research pursuits are very different, however, and often attract different kinds of people who engage in them.

When Allen Steere arrived in New Haven in July 1975 as a first-year fellow in rheumatology at the Yale medical school, he was required to develop a research project. He had already completed an internship and residency in internal medicine and had spent an additional two years working with the CDC in Atlanta as an EIS officer in the hospital infections branch. Now, in New Haven, he was doing some clinical work and had also just started a bench research project that involved examining the tiny granules in polymorphonuclear leukocytes, a kind of white blood cell that fights infections. Steere wasn't opposed to doing bench research, but his heart wasn't in this particular project. With the developments in the Lyme area, however, his life was about to change.

"I remember three things happening very close to the same time," Steere recalls. "And it was the fact that multiple things happened at the same time that was most compelling, as opposed to any one of those events by itself. I remember Mrs. Mensch's call, and she was very articulate. So you got a very clear picture of what she was telling you, that her daughter had acquired an illness . . . that had been diagnosed as JRA. And then very close in time, I heard from Bob Gifford, who was a faculty member in the rheumatology division, that he was scheduled to see a woman from Lyme, Connecticut, who had arthritis and in fact, that her whole family had arthritis. And at the same time, David Snydman also called saying that he was looking into this too."

Snydman and Steere knew each other from their days in Atlanta with the CDC. Snydman told Steere about the phone calls from Mrs. Murray (on October 16) and from Mrs. Mensch (about two weeks later) and that he had been checking into the situation in the Lyme area. Snydman also told his former colleague that he was planning

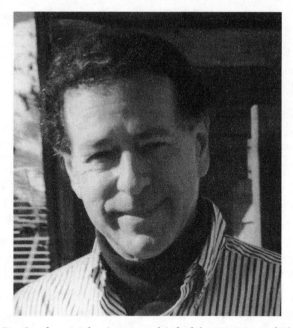

Figure 4. Dr. Stephen Malawista was chief of the Division of Rheumatology at Yale University in the mid-1970s, when doctors at Yale began investigating Lyme disease. (Photo from the mid-1970s, courtesy of Stephen Malawista, M.D.)

to investigate further and asked whether Steere would be interested in joining him in his investigations. Dr. Stephen Malawista (Figure 4) was the chief of the Division of Rheumatology at Yale at the time and Steere's direct supervisor. Upon hearing the news, he remembers looking up whether JRA had been reported previously in clusters. It had not. He and Steere also calculated the expected incidence of JRA in the three towns of Lyme, Old Lyme, and East Haddam. On the basis of a population for the three towns of twelve thousand individuals, the expected number of cases was one! It was unheard of for JRA to cluster like it seemed to be doing in the Lyme area.

"I could conceive of a rubella [German measles] outbreak where multiple people would have arthritis," Steere recalls, "but that was something that they could rule out fairly quickly. If it wasn't rubella, it [the clustering] had never been described with JRA and I felt it was

Yale - New Haven Medical Center

DANA DIAGNOSTIC CENTER
DANA III
789 HOWARD AVE., NEW HAVEN, CT. 06504
(203) 436–8060

Polly Murray

Your appointment with

Dr. **Robert H. Gifford**   (Rheumatology)

is on_____ **Thursday, November 20, 1975 at 1:30 p.m.**

Should you be unable to keep this appointment, please let us know immediately as other patients are waiting for appointments.

Figure 5. Polly Murray's appointment card at Yale–New Haven Medical Center, November 20, 1975. She met with Dr. Allen Steere, who was also looking into "what was happening in Lyme." (Courtesy of Polly Murray.)

very important to look into the situation. David [Snydman] invited me to come over as he had scheduled some time to see some of the children in the local health department. And I also told Bob Gifford that I would very much like to see Polly Murray. And she came over."

On Thursday, November 20, 1975, Mrs. Murray drove down Route 95 to her appointment at Yale (Figure 5). She remembers being surprised, and a little put off at first, when the young Dr. Steere sat down to speak with her rather than Dr. Gifford. This is standard procedure at most academic teaching hospitals, however, and Steere's open, curious manner quickly put her at ease. By this point, Steere had already communicated with Snydman and had spoken with Mrs. Mensch, so it was not just Polly Murray's personal case he was looking into, but the whole phenomenon of "what was happening in Lyme."

Polly Murray's visit with Dr. Steere was not typical of a doctor's appointment in several ways. For one, it lasted more than three hours. Also, the doctor did most of the listening and the patient most of the talking. By this time, Mrs. Murray had compiled a list of more than thirty-five people whom she believed were having similar problems. With their permission, she had recorded the case histories and catalogued their lab tests and consultations. "She brought her notebook," Steere recalls, "and started telling me about her family members, and she had catalogued what each of them had had and her own experience, as well as the experiences of various people who lived in the area. And I listened."

Polly Murray later wrote: "He asked me to start at the beginning. Right away I was struck by his openness. He was understanding and unhurried in his approach. I didn't feel that I had to rush through sentences; here was a doctor who was ready to listen, who was genuinely interested in the story. He took notes as I talked; I gave him a copy of my medical history, and we carefully went over the outlines I had written up for Dr. Schur, detailing all the symptoms that each of us had."

Toward the end of the appointment, Drs. Gifford and Malawista entered the room. Mrs. Murray recalls sensing a feeling of excitement in the air, as if the doctors felt that this was truly a phenomenon worthy of investigation. Finally, she had conveyed her story to people who listened and who would try to do something about it.

At this point, Steere, Malawista, and Snydman began planning how to best go about investigating "what was happening in Lyme." From the beginning, Malawista, realizing that the laboratory experiments did not seem to hold much passion for the young Steere, generously supported Steere. Also, Malawista recalls that early in the sequence of events, he had a feeling that they were on the verge of something important: "It was pretty early that I realized that this is an infectious disease that is acting like an inflammatory rheumatic disease. That was its major interest to me. Because in rheumatology, I've always thought that if we were only smarter we'd be part of infectious diseases because we'd know what the organisms were that were at least triggering the [joint] disease. They are triggered by something, and chances are it's infectious. And here was a disease that by its clustering—it was clustering in time, it was clustering in space, it was clustering in families and on roads—it really looked like there was a vector [something that transmits the disease, such as an insect]."

Arthritis caused by direct bacterial invasion is called a *septic arthritis* or a septic joint. Patients with septic arthritis generally look sick and feel sick. They usually have a fever. The joint is typically red, warm, and tender. In a typical septic joint, many tens of thousands of white blood cells are found per cubic centimeter of fluid, and sometimes, obvious pus. Also, bacteria can be cultured from the fluid. What intrigued Malawista was something altogether different, far more subtle, and potentially far more significant: the possibility that an infectious agent was causing not an overtly infected joint but an inflamed joint. It appeared that some sort of infection was triggering inflammation in the joint, and that once the inflammation got started, it took on a life of its own.

The notion that an infectious organism could cause a disease that was not classically considered to be of infectious origin was not entirely new in the mid-1970s. In fact, one disease, rheumatic fever—which some of Polly Murray's doctors considered as her diagnosis at one point—is a model of this phenomenon. Rheumatic fever is an inflammatory disease that is a complication of streptococcal infection in the throat, or strep throat. More specifically, following a pharyngitis (inflamed throat) with specific strains of strep (group A, beta-hemolytic), various, and at times bizarre, patterns of inflammation can occur in several parts of the body—especially the heart, joints, and skin. The disease follows stages; after the acute sore throat, patients improve for several weeks and then may develop a baffling array of symptoms.

The arthritis they get is of the oligoarticular variety and tends to migrate from one large joint to the next. Many patients develop inflammation of the heart as well. The lining of the heart including the valves, the muscle of the heart, as well as the outer sac—the pericardium—in which the heart sits, all become inflamed. Some patients develop odd rashes that come and go; others manifest nodules in the skin, especially over bony surfaces and over joints. Some patients are left with their arms flailing about uncontrollably and purposeless, in a neurological manifestation called Sydenham's chorea, or St. Vitus's dance.

Most patients heal and do well over the ensuing weeks to months, but some are left with serious incompetence or tightening of the cardiac valves, a problem that may endure through their lifetimes and ultimately be treatable only with surgical intervention. The incidence of rheumatic fever has fallen in North America over the past sixty years. In the 1940s, the incidence was 65 cases, mostly school-aged children, per 100,000 of population. In 1978, that number plunged to 9 per 100,000, and it was even lower at the century mark. How much of this decrease is attributable to antibiotic use in patients with strep throat, how much to overall improvements in public health and hygiene, and how much to other factors related to the streptococcal strains is unclear; however, two observations are clear: the incidence of a disease may increase or decrease precipitously over relatively short periods of time, and rheumatic fever still exists and physicians see cases from time to time.

Rheumatic fever provides us with another piece of important information. Doctors use the term *pathogenesis* to designate how a disease occurs; that is, on a cellular or molecular level, what is actually happening to the tissues to produce the signs and symptoms? In rheumatic fever, the initial strep infection leads to inflammation in distant parts of the body. Why does this happen? It is because some portions of the cell surface on particular streptococci display a landscape, a topography, that is very much like the topography on some cells of the body—heart cells, for example. So as the patient's immune system mounts its offense against the invading streptococcus, the antibodies formed sometimes cannot tell the difference between the invading bacteria that they are meant to kill and the host heart cell, which looks very similar.

It's simply a case of mistaken identity. If the police put out an APB on a medium-height white male wearing a tan coat and black hat, they may round up ten men who meet that general description. But they won't be identical. Some might have tan coats, others beige jackets. One might have a dark gray bowler hat; another, a jet-black Stetson; still another, a Yankees baseball cap. Similarly, antibodies can sometimes be fooled by this molecular mimicry.

The notion that an infection can trigger an inflammatory illness has become even more common over time. Perhaps the best example is inflammation of the stomach (gastritis) and peptic ulcers. When in the early 1980s Dr. Barry Marshall published his initial work on this idea in the prestigious British medical journal *Lancet,* the article met with enormous skepticism. The prevailing wisdom was that too much acid in the stomach caused ulcers. Other factors such as stress, spicy foods, hormones, smoking, and alcohol were thought to play roles. Surgery for ulcers was commonplace. The now widely known fact that bacteria caused ulcers was thought preposterous at the time. And that time was not very long ago.

The concept of infection leading to inflammation is not limited to diseases of the stomach. Some believe that chlamydial infection leads to coronary artery disease and heart attacks. Prions, a novel class of infectious material, are thought to cause the feared bovine spongiform encephalitis, or mad cow disease. Some data suggest that hepatitis C virus is related to liver cancer and that human papilloma virus causes cervical cancer.

But pinning down the specific cause and defining the pathology were not the first order of business for Dr. Snydman and the men from Yale. They first needed to organize and direct an investigation so that, if nature was providing them with other clues about how the disease worked, they would be ready to find them. The fact that this seemed to be a phenomenon never before described only heightened their excitement and sense of purpose. And so they carefully planned an investigation of this outbreak of arthritis.

5 • An Outbreak of Arthritis

As David Snydman began examining children in the Lyme area and speaking to local physicians to get a better idea of how common the problem was, more and more dots appeared on his map, each representing a case of arthritis. Early in the investigation, Dr. Steere had had the opportunity to examine the entire Murray family. "That was very telling because when you examined each one individually," he recalls, "not every family member was affected, but there were three family members who were all affected at the same time. They had swelling of the knees; they had an inflammatory arthritis. So it [the pattern] was very clear.

"It was also clear when you saw all three of them that their clinical history did not fit anything previously described. But they seemed very legitimate. I mean, they could describe articulately what they had observed. So I told Dr. Malawista that I had seen them and I went to Lyme to see these other teenagers who had arthritis. I really wanted to work on it." Malawista and Steere agreed that Steere would devote the next six months to analyzing the mysterious cluster of children from the Lyme area who had arthritis.

But an investigation such as this needs far more focus and organization than simply having a few doctors drive around the community trying to find patients with swollen knees. To study this phenomenon properly, they needed to be able to put a label on it, to define it so that they could separate the "it" from everything else that was going on in the Lyme area. They needed what John Snow already had in his cholera victims—a *case definition*. For a variety of reasons, the arthritis was selected as the central part of the case definition. For one thing, the doctors from Yale who planned the investigation were rheumatologists—specialists who study arthritis. So it was natural for them to focus on the joint manifestations. Second, the arthritis was clearly a central part of the mystery. Although rashes had been described in some patients and Mrs. Murray had suffered various neurological symptoms, the most prominent manifestation was swelling and inflammation of the joints. In addition, a swollen joint was something that would not be expected to occur very frequently by chance, especially in children.

Snydman and Steere, with Malawista closely supervising, wrote a protocol for evaluating this outbreak of arthritis (Figure 6). The two younger physicians had just spent significant time at the CDC doing just this—evaluating outbreaks of disease; they knew the drill. And so with their simple case definition—children in the Lyme area with arthritis—they set about finding cases. They first had to clear the investigation with the Yale Human Investigations Committee. This committee, sometimes called an Institutional Review Board, is composed of a group of people, generally both doctors and laypeople, whose purpose is to decide whether research that investigators are planning at that medical center sufficiently protects the safety and privacy of the patients who are subjects. Dr. Steere spent a fair amount of time and effort writing the protocol, which was approved by the committee at Yale.

Protocol 1125 consisted of first identifying children with arthritis in the three contiguous communities of Old Lyme, Lyme, and East Haddam, Connecticut. This proved fairly easy. Investigators spoke with local doctors, school nurses, and health officials as well as perhaps their greatest source of information—the patients that Mrs. Mensch and Mrs. Murray had unofficially identified. They also pored over discharge diagnosis lists from local hospitals, looking for JRA or

Protocol for Clinical Research Study

Yale University School of Medicine

Yale-New Haven Hospital

Date___December 1, 1975___

Title of Project

Evaluation of Epidemic Arthritis in the Lyme, Connecticut area

Chief Investigator   Allen C. Steere[1]

Other Investigators   Stephen E. Malawista,[1] Warren Andiman,[2] Philip Askenase,[3] Robert Shope[4]
Dorothy Horstmann,[2,4] and David Snydman[5]

School Department (or Departments)

Department of Internal Medicine/Rheumatology[1]
Department of Internal Medicine/Clinical Immunology[3]
Department of Pediatrics[2]
Dept. of Epidemiology and Public Health[4]
Connecticut State Health Department[5]

Department Chairman   Samuel O. Thier, M.D[1]

Chairman/Pediatrics   Howard A. Pearson, M.D

(space below this line for Clinical Investigation Committee use)

_____   _____
Date Approved   Clinical Investigation Committee, Chairman

_____   _____
Date Approved   Clinical Research Center, Director

Interim approval granted
15 December 1975
Thomas C. Chalmers, M.D

Figure 6. First page of the protocol for the original study of the patients in Lyme, showing the names of the investigators and departments involved and approval handwritten in the lower left. (Courtesy of David Snydman, M.D.)

other diagnoses of arthritis in children. The official period of the study ranged from December 1975 through May 1976.

The investigators offered to the patients a full evaluation at the Yale rheumatology clinic but were careful to do so through local doctors and health clinics so that it did not appear as if the big academic medical center was trying to scoop away their patients—a common conflict between private practitioners in a community and doctors at a large academic medical center. Thus, the children were invited to travel to Yale to be examined so that other causes of arthritis could be excluded. Over the next six months, Steere would examine all of the identified patients. In his examination, he would take an exhaustive medical history, perform a physical examination, and have blood drawn to be tested later for numerous known pathogens. If there were fluid in the joint at the time of the examination, he would perform a synovial biopsy. *Synovium,* the tissue that lines our joints, can be sampled by a special kind of needle with a tiny hook on its side. At the same time that the doctor performs an arthrocentesis, using this special needle, he can take a sample of the synovial tissue as well.

Other members of the team contacted the other physicians who had seen the patients at the height of their illnesses—general practitioners, internists, pediatricians, rheumatologists, orthopedic surgeons, and ophthalmologists—to obtain more information.

The Yale group identified fifty-one patients who met their inclusion criteria: thirty-nine children and twelve adults. When viewed as a group, a clear pattern began to emerge. The arthritis typically began suddenly; the knee was most frequently involved, followed by the wrist, ankle, and temporomandibular joint (where the jaw meets the skull). The pattern of joint involvement was monoarticular in 69 percent and oligoarticular in 29 percent of patients; only a single patient had polyarticular involvement. The duration of arthritis was typically short, only about one week, but lasted for as long as six months in some patients. Some of the patients initially improved, only to suffer from recurrences later. Furthermore, even when patients had severely swollen joints, they often experienced little pain. When the investigators analyzed the children separately from the adults, there were no differences, suggesting that all suffered from the same malady.

More than half of the patients reported other symptoms such as fever, malaise and fatigue, headache, and muscle pains. A few had a nondescript rash. Seven of the twelve adults suffered from profound fatigue and had bizarre sensory symptoms that persisted for months after the arthritis had gone. One crucial observation was a negative one. None of the children had inflammation of the front portion of the eye (iritis), a symptom that would have been expected if they did in fact have JRA.

Perhaps the most important finding of the study was that thirteen of the patients (25 percent) had a red, circular or ring-shaped lesion, often on their legs or arms, that became eight to twenty inches in diameter in some patients. Some described concentric red rings, separated by normal appearing skin—like a bull's-eye. Some patients had more than one lesion. Some had fever, severe headache, or stiff neck associated with the lesion. One even experienced paralysis of half of the face. Many of the patients and their physicians thought the rash to be secondary to an insect bite, but only one patient remembered being bitten at the site of the rash—in that case, by a tick.

Equally important to the identification of this unusual rash was the epidemiological analysis. The three communities that formed the basis of the study were all situated along the eastern bank of the Connecticut River. Old Lyme also bordered on Long Island Sound. The investigators looked for what the patients had in common. At one point, they suspected the water supply, but each of the households had its own well. The children from Lyme and Old Lyme shared a school system, but those from East Haddam had their own.

Besides the general location of the communities affected, the investigators found other geographical clustering. None of the affected patients lived in the town centers, living instead in more rural areas. In fact, even within the small towns, geographical clustering was marked. Half of the affected residents from Old Lyme and East Haddam lived on just a few adjoining roads. "On some streets, it was one house after another," Steere says. "I can't tell you how different that is from JRA. I had been given a list of names to telephone. Once I dialed the wrong number and got a home where that child had arthritis!"

The investigators also confirmed what Snydman had known from the beginning—that the onset of symptoms was tightly clustered seasonally. For the most part, the arthritis tended to develop in patients during late summer and early fall, and all of the patients who experienced the rash did so from June through September. Another clue was that when neighbors or members of the same family fell ill, they frequently did so in different years. This pattern was also true for other people who knew one another, such as classmates.

The investigators searched for other common circumstances but found none. What was the common thread? The people affected didn't swim in the same pool or lake. They didn't eat the same food. There was no common history of immunizations. Many of the patients had pet ownership in common, but this was not at all unusual in the area.

The laboratory testing on the samples of blood and joint fluid also were unrevealing. The joint fluid did not grow out any bacteria. The amounts of white blood cells and the types of cells varied considerably from patient to patient. Chemical analysis of the blood and joint fluid was similarly unrewarding. Finally, X rays of the affected joints and microscopic examination of the tissue taken from the synovial biopsies that Steere performed were equally nondiagnostic.

Nevertheless, the investigators were able to reach several conclusions, as well as devise a plan to further attack the problem. With the advantage of having the forest to examine, rather than just the trees, they were able to dispel the notion that the children were suffering from JRA. First, the pattern of joint involvement was wrong. All of the patients had monoarticular or oligoarticular arthritis, whereas only about 40 percent of patients with JRA show this pattern. Second, when JRA patients do have the oligoarticular pattern, there is a female-to-male ratio of three to one and age peaks of one to three and nine to eleven years. The patients in the Lyme area had no marked predisposition to girls, and the ages of the patients also did not fit the pattern. Certainly, JRA is extraordinarily rare in adults, and twelve of the fifty-one patients—nearly a quarter—were adults. Third, as noted above, none of the Lyme children suffered from iritis, which a proportion of patients with JRA would be expected to have. JRA patients also have certain kinds of autoantibodies in their blood, which the Lyme cohort did not exhibit.

The next line of evidence was the duration of joint swelling. Many of the patients from Connecticut had very brief episodes of joint swelling, whereas those with JRA typically suffer from much longer episodes of pain and swelling. If one had applied specific criteria that were used in the mid-1970s to diagnose JRA, only between 30 and 50 percent of the patients would have met them.

The most compelling argument against the JRA diagnoses, however, was the clustering. Juvenile rheumatoid arthritis simply had never been known to cluster in time, in space, and in families. The arthritis cases were clustering at about one hundred times the expected prevalence of JRA in this community. Nearly every family had at least one child affected. The likelihood of this happening purely by chance was remote.

The patterns of geographical and seasonal clustering strongly suggested to the investigators that they were dealing with a vector-borne disease, most likely a virus transmitted by an insect.

Humans become diseased in only so many ways. A genetic defect in an enzyme may result in the production of a faulty protein, which can cause a given syndrome. Trauma can break a bone or tear a blood vessel. Eating food or drinking water that has been tainted with a poison or a microorganism can cause various ailments. Too much or too little of something in the diet, such as calcium or sodium, can lead to serious illness.

Some diseases are vector-borne. The word *vector* derives from the Latin *vectus,* which means "bearer" or "carrier." Therefore, in its medical usage, the word refers to any organism that is the carrier of a disease-producing agent. Many vectors of human disease are from one of two classes of arthropods—insects and arachnids. Arthropod-borne viruses are called *arboviruses.* Of the insects, mosquitoes are probably the most notorious vector for arboviruses, but flies, fleas, lice, and other bugs transmit a variety of maladies all over the world. For example, the tsetse fly is the vector for African sleeping sickness, a protozoan disease caused by the organism *Trypanasoma brucei gambiense.* The flea is the vector for the bubonic plague bacillus, the bacteria that decimated much of Europe in the fourteenth century. Lice are vectors for the dread typhus fever. Of the arachnids, ticks are the most important vectors, although mites also contribute.

Perhaps the most notorious of all vector-borne diseases and the most common worldwide is malaria—a treatable infection that is a common cause of childhood mortality in some parts of the world. Tiny organisms called protozoa are transmitted by the bite of an infected mosquito to susceptible humans. But mosquitoes can transmit various classes of microorganisms besides protozoa, including viruses, bacteria, and tiny worms. Some of the viruses are known to cause epidemic arthritis.

Chikungunya fever is one. The name derives from a word in an east African dialect meaning "that which bends up." Mosquitoes can spread this virus to humans; at times, enormous epidemics have occurred, including one that affected more than twenty million people in Indonesia in the mid-1980s. The responsible virus was isolated in Tanzania in 1950 and continues to plague the inhabitants of Africa and Asia. Chikungunya fever causes abrupt onset of fever, headache, and muscle and joint pains—some of the same symptoms seen in the Connecticut outbreak. But the joint involvement is usually symmetric (for example, it affects both knees or both elbows). It also affects adults worse than children. Furthermore, a nondescript rash— many tiny red spots and bumps—occurs in three-quarters of patients, something not seen in the Lyme patients. Also, the white blood cell and platelet counts tend to be low, another finding that was absent in the Lyme outbreak.

Another mosquito-borne virus known to cause arthritis has an equally strange name—o'nyong-nyong—which means "weakening in the joints" in a Ugandan dialect. This disease primarily occurs in sub-Saharan Africa and produces symptoms and laboratory findings similar to those of Chikungunya fever.

The last mosquito-borne disease known to cause arthritis is Ross River disease, which occurs in Australia. The symptoms are similar to those of the other two diseases. The arthritis is usually polyarticular and tends to symmetrically involve smaller joints such as the wrists, ankles, and small joints of the hands and feet. It, too, is associated with a rash, but again, one that is not typical of the large expanding area of erythema, or redness, seen in the patients in coastal Connecticut.

Yale was uniquely equipped to test for arboviruses because Dr. Robert E. Shope, a member of the staff there, was a world authority on them and maintained an arbovirus reference laboratory. In fact, the Yale researchers tested for Chikungunya, o'nyong-nyong, and Ross River disease viruses, as well as for more than one hundred other microorganisms, including bacteria, viruses, rickettsiae, leptospira, and mycoplasma.

Dr. Warren Andiman, who was just finishing his training in pediatric infectious diseases as well as viral diagnosis, led much of the search for a virus. Viruses are not easy to see. In the mid-1970s, most viral diagnostic work was done with tissue culture and serology. This meant taking some of the blood or joint fluid from the patients Dr. Steere was seeing in the clinic and injecting it onto layers of cells in the laboratory to see whether unseen viruses might be damaging the cells—a so-called *cytopathic effect.*

Andiman remembers: "The rheumatologists sent us specimens—joint fluid and sometimes synovial biopsies—to try to find a viral etiology. As we got more and more specimens, I became interested in finding out who these patients were. And so I asked Allen if I could come to the clinic to see who these patients were, to get a graphic impression, a clinical impression, in the hope that perhaps something in clinical appearance or history would help us decide how to tailor the lab part to better help. So I started being an observer with Allen. I remember on occasion when he did a joint tap, I would take the specimens and then do the inoculation. We accumulated racks and racks of tissue culture tubes to look for cytopathic effects."

But despite this extensive laboratory effort, neither any of the routine laboratory tests nor anything from the sophisticated labs of either Shope or Andiman revealed anything suspicious.

The investigators also tested for another infectious cause of epidemic arthritis—one not quite as exotic as the arboviruses that Shope's lab was seeking. In fact, large epidemics of this kind of arthritis had occurred at least twice before in the United States, one of them in New England. This epidemic erupted much like that of Snow's cholera. The first case occurred on January 2, 1926, in the industrial town of Haverhill, Massachusetts. A few cases appeared two days later, and then starting on the eleventh of the month, multiple cases began showing up every day—as many as eleven in a single day.

Patients developed abrupt onset of fever, chills, headache, vomiting, and rash. Most of them also developed an acute polyarthritis involving multiple small and large joints. Local health officials, with help from experts in Boston, did the same kind of case mapping that Snow had done seventy-five years before and that Snydman did fifty years after that. The map revealed that all of the cases were tightly clustered in a small rectangle of town bordered by the Merrimack River. No association with specific foods was found, nor with the water supply, nor with outside plumbing (all affected houses had indoor privies). However, all of the patients bought their milk from the same dairy or from stores that bought their milk from that dairy. The dairy was a small, family-run operation that priced their milk a penny less per quart than their competition. They could underprice because they skipped the pasteurizing process.

The organism that was cultured out of the blood from some of the patients was *Streptobacillus moniliformis*, the agent that causes rat-bite fever. This microorganism is commonly found in rats and is usually transmitted through the bite of a rat into the skin. The bacteria can also be introduced through the gut. The manner of contamination in this outbreak was never determined; however, on January 27, the milk was ordered pasteurized and the epidemic vanished. To this day, rat-bite fever is sometimes referred to as Haverhill fever.

The Yale investigators tested for antibodies to this organism as well, and again came up empty handed. But they felt fairly confident of three things, at this point. First, they were not dealing with JRA. Second, they were quite certain that they were dealing with a new, as yet unrecognized disease. And third, on the basis of the information they had at the end of their initial study period, they believed that the cause of this new entity was a vector-borne virus.

6 • An Outbreak of Dermatitis

The southern coast of Connecticut stretches along Long Island Sound. That portion of the coast between New Haven to the west and Watch Hill, Rhode Island, to the east runs directly east-west. Two large rivers punctuate that coastline—the Connecticut River at Old Lyme and the Thames River at New London, approximately sixteen miles away from one another. Slightly upriver and on the eastern bank of the Thames, the New London Naval Submarine Base occupies approximately five hundred acres and has more than four hundred buildings, which include the housing and support facilities for ten thousand active-duty and civilian workers and their families. Because of the number of both enlisted men and their families, the base boasts a medical facility staffed by Navy doctors—the Submarine Medical Center, in Groton. In 1975, two of the twenty-five or so Navy doctors stationed there were confronted by a case that was unique in their professional careers.

It was peak summer—months before Mrs. Mensch and Mrs. Murray placed their calls to the Connecticut State Health Department—when a seventy-three-year-old man walked into the office of Lieutenant Commander William Mast (Figure 7), an internist at the base, to consult with him about an odd rash. A couple of weeks before

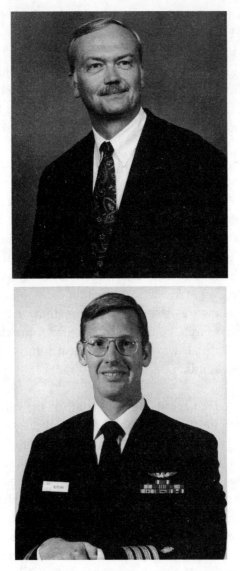

Figure 7. Lieutenant Commander William Mast, M.D., and Commander William Burrows, M.D., were doctors at the Naval Submarine Medical Center in Groton, Connecticut, when they saw a patient in 1976 with a large rash on his thigh and torso, later determined to be erythema migrans (EM) and associated with Lyme disease. (Courtesy of William Mast, M.D., and William Burrows, M.D.)

the appointment, the patient had noticed a small red itchy patch on his left thigh. He had initially assumed that it was due to some unknown insect bite, but over the ensuing weeks, the rash continued to grow. The ringlike eruption eventually got so big that the patient sought a medical opinion. Mast had never seen such a large area of erythema (redness), which had spread from the man's thigh onto his torso. Fortunately, a dermatologist was on base with whom he could consult on such cases.

Commander William Burrows was only thirty-two years old in 1974 when he received his first commission at the Submarine Medical Center, where he performed all dermatology consults for the sailors, retirees, and their dependents who were referred to him. Burrows was impressed by what he saw on the patient Mast had referred. The erythema had grown to be about the diameter of a large cantaloupe and was simultaneously itchy and tender. "The guy was in excellent health, but felt kind of lousy, with mild flulike symptoms," Burrows recalls. "All I knew was that this was something I had never seen before. I couldn't easily culture it, but it was somewhat tender. So based on that, I decided to empirically treat him [with antibiotics] as if it were a cellulitis."

Cellulitis, which means inflammation of the cells, is the term doctors use for infection of the skin. Like the heart or the pancreas, the skin is actually an organ and provides vital functions for us. It helps maintain normal temperature and fluid homeostasis in the body. Patients with severe burns, for example, require enormous amounts of intravenous fluids to keep them from becoming dangerously dehydrated. Another important function of the skin is keeping the "outside world"—specifically, bacteria and other microorganisms—outside. Bacteria on the surface of our skin may exist as contaminants or carriers, but they are unlikely to wreck havoc unless they gain access to the tissues beneath the outer layer. Normally, this occurs because of a minor trauma, such as a rose thorn piercing the outer layer of skin or epidermis or a nail puncturing the sole of the foot. Sometimes, microorganisms might mount a coordinated, synchronized attack. For instance, the fungus responsible for athlete's foot may cause enough irritation or inflammation so that streptococ-cal bacteria, normally minding their own business on the skin's sur-face, have a portal of entry into the body.

Once bacteria penetrate the skin, which is our first, outer perim-eter of defense, they may begin to multiply or produce toxins in the immediate area. Or they may gain access to other parts of the body by hitching a ride via lymph channels or blood vessels. In establishing themselves in the skin, the bacteria must multiply because one lonely staphylococcus or streptococcus will not survive long against the host of defense mechanisms the body will launch. White blood cells of various classes, antibodies specifically tailored and manufactured for a given species of bacteria, and other plasma proteins will be signaled to travel to the area to combat the invaders. Blood vessels dilate to accommodate the increased cellular and molecular traffic, and these vessels become more permeable so that the advanced guard can gain access to the front lines of battle. The patient notices the cardinal signs of inflammation—redness, warmth, pain, and swelling.

Cellulitis most commonly occurs where trauma to the skin most commonly occurs—on the extremities. But cellulitis on the thigh is unusual. Also, cellulitis usually is painful, especially as it grows in-creasingly large. Furthermore, patients with a large cellulitis often have a fever, and they generally look and feel unwell.

The red rash of Burrows and Mast's patient didn't fit into any well-known pattern. Several factors about the rash—its size, location, duration, minor amount of pain—made them question the diagnosis. But because it might have been an atypical cellulitis, they thought it might respond to antibiotics. Without articulating that he was per-forming a "therapeutic trial," that is precisely what Burrows did. He administered oral antibiotics—250 milligrams of erythromycin four times per day. And as one must do for any therapeutic trial, he re-examined the patient a couple of days later. The rash had vanished, and the Navy doctors concluded that the erythromycin had cured whatever the rash was. The patient was treated for seven days and did not have any subsequent recurrences during the three months of careful follow-up care. The patient was better, and that was that.

But that wasn't that. During one month, three other patients with the same kind of unusual erythema appeared. One was a thirty-three-year-old man with high fevers, severe malaise, and a large red rash on his right shoulder. During his illness, the man's eight-year-old son also developed a similar advancing ring of erythema on his body, and he, too, had fever and soreness in the muscles. Another young man, twenty-one years old, developed the same kind of rash, this time on the calf. With this fourth case, Burrows obtained a small piece of tissue to study the microscopic architecture of this strange erythema. He found many white blood cells (lymphocytes) clustered around the blood vessels in the tissue specimen, but this nonspecific finding did not allow him to make any particular diagnosis.

But Burrows did another thing. Each Wednesday morning, he drove along the coast to New Haven so that he could participate in the grand rounds of the Department of Dermatology at Yale University School of Medicine.

Doctors participate in different kinds of rounds. During daily hospital rounds, doctors visit their hospitalized patients, usually in the early morning, to check on progress, review test results, and speak with the patients. In academic teaching hospitals, these rounds are often called *work rounds. Grand rounds* are more formal and have an educational focus. Years ago during grand rounds, experienced physicians would interact with a patient in the lecture hall, taking the patient's history and performing as much of a physical examination as could be done with propriety. The doctor would then discuss the diagnostic and therapeutic possibilities related to the patient's problem. Over time, this exercise gradually evolved into a lecture by senior physicians in a particular area or perhaps by a visiting professor. Sometimes, doctors would present interesting cases or diagnostic dilemmas.

Twenty-five years ago, in an era that afforded private physicians if not more leisure time, at least more control over it, doctors would frequently break from the routine of their day to attend these grand rounds to keep abreast of the latest advances in medicine. So in 1975, each Wednesday morning, Bill Burrows was in the habit of attending Yale dermatology grand rounds. Sometimes the doctors would present interesting cases or diagnostic dilemmas. Burrows took this opportunity to present his cases of the odd rashes from Groton. He orally presented the case histories and then showed pictures of the rashes and the biopsy specimen. One of the doctors in the group, Dr. Thomas Hansen, commented that these rashes sounded very much like something that had been reported in Europe many decades ago—a rash called erythema chronicum migrans (ECM).

"By sheer chance," Hansen recalls, "I had been reading something recently in a journal, I think the *Archives [of Dermatology]*, about ECM in Europe and I said it sounded the same. It wasn't any kind of 'eureka' or anything. I remembered it occurred in Sweden and was associated with an arthropod or something."

Hansen may have been referring to a case report by Dr. Rudolph Scrimenti (Figure 8), a dermatologist practicing in Milwaukee, Wisconsin, published in the *Archives of Dermatology* in 1970. The patient was a fifty-seven-year-old physician who spent a great deal of time outdoors hunting grouse. His chief complaint was of a large expanding erythema on his right chest and torso that had started at the site of a tick bite. Like many physicians who become patients, he had already tried treating himself, with a topical steroid that had not helped. Scrimenti biopsied the rash and had found the same nonspecific findings that Burrows had found—lymphocytes around blood vessels.

For Scrimenti, seeing that patient *was* a moment of "eureka." As a medical student, he had read a paper about ECM by Dr. Sven Hellerstrom, a Swedish dermatologist, whose work was reprinted in the *Southern Journal of Medicine* in 1950. Several years later Scrimenti wrote in the *Wisconsin Medical Journal* that that paper first caught his attention when he was a medical student around 1958 because Hellerstrom's findings showed "the possibility of diagnosing, and perhaps even treating multi-system disorders on the basis of observable skin manifestations. As I was yet undecided as to which medical specialty I would enter, Dr. Hellerstrom's description of the visual detective work involved in diagnosing patients with ECM with meningitis influenced my decision to go into dermatology. It also kept me on the lookout for similar cases."

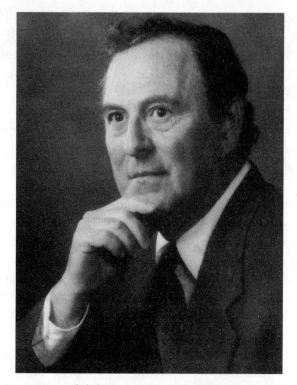

Figure 8. In 1970, Rudolph Scrimenti, M.D., reported on the first case of erythema migrans (EM) in North America and treated it successfully with penicillin, as had European doctors before him. (Courtesy of Rudolph Scrimenti, M.D.)

And so in 1970, Scrimenti, who had been searching for a case for twelve years, finally made the diagnosis of ECM, the first case ever documented in the United States (Figure 9). Being well-versed in the European literature of the time that showed the benefit of antibiotics, Scrimenti promptly treated his patient with penicillin. The patient improved and remained free of recurrences for the next twenty years.

Mast and Burrows decided to write up their four cases of ECM because of their significance. "To the best of our knowledge," they wrote in the *Journal of the American Medical Association (JAMA)* in August 1976, "this is the first appearance of a cluster of cases of ECM in the United States. Our cases illustrate the varying degrees of sys-

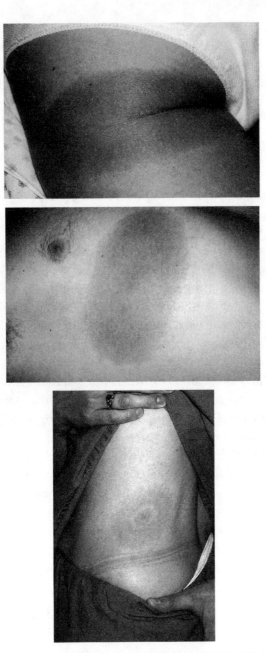

Figure 9. Three patients with erythema migrans (EM). (Photographs by Jonathan Edlow, M.D.)

temic involvement, ranging from a minimally symptomatic chronic progressive skin lesion to a generalized severe illness." They went on to write, "The occurrence of multiple cases of ECM within a limited geographical area within a one-month period lends further support to the concept of an infectious and insect-borne etiology." The two Navy doctors concluded: "Although this cluster of cases may be a solitary and unique occurrence, it is possible that further incidence of this previously rare disease will ensue with the following summer season. We hope this report will result in the widespread recognition of this disease by physicians in the United States."

This is precisely what happened for Dr. Edgar Grunwaldt, a family practitioner on Shelter Island—a small island couched between the north and south forks of Long Island at the latter's eastern tip. "I came to Shelter Island in the summer of 1975," Grunwaldt recalls. "I believe that I got here on May 30. I began seeing patients with what I thought were infected insect bites—big red blotches, and being from New York City, I had never seen them before." He treated them with penicillin. The next spring and summer, Grunwaldt saw even more cases.

Then in August of 1976, when Mast and Burrows published their article in *JAMA*, Grunwaldt, too, experienced a moment of "eureka." "I remembered the report by the navy doctors in *JAMA*," Grunwaldt says, "and then I found an old dermatology textbook we had at the hospital and looked up ECM (erythema chronicum migrans) and found that it had been described in Europe. In fact, there was someone, I cannot remember his name, who thought that it was a spirochete [a kind of bacterium] which he got from tissue samples. He inoculated himself and [discovered] the fact that penicillin seemed to work. That had been written up in Europe in the '40s."

Several lines of evidence kept pointing to Europe.

7 • The European Connection

What was the history of this rash—which several doctors in the United States suspected they were seeing—in Europe?

At the 1909 meeting of the Swedish Dermatological Society in Stockholm, a prominent dermatologist, Arvid Afzelius, presented a case of an older woman with a gradually enlarging red rash that followed the bite of the European sheep tick, *Ixodes ricinus*. During those days, dermatology was just becoming a specialty unto itself, and many of the practitioners of dermatology were specialists in syphilis. Thus the case report was recorded in the journal *Archiv fur Dermatologie und Syphilis* in 1910. His patient's rash started at the site of the bite and then slowly expanded centrifugally, clearing in the center as it did so—again, something like a bull's-eye. Afzelius was the first to use the term *erythema migrans* (EM) to describe this never-before-reported skin eruption. The following year, Wilhelm Balban of Vienna described three cases of an annular erythema following insect bites although he never specified which insect was responsible.

Then in 1913, another Viennese physician recorded another case of an annular erythema, this time in a twenty-nine-year-old woman. It began as a red spot on the back of her left thigh and migrated onto her buttock and leg over many months, completely resolving only after seven months. To emphasize the chronic nature of this patient's case, the physician, Benjamin Lipschutz, called the rash erythema *chronicum* migrans (ECM).

Lipschutz published his account in the same journal as both Afzelius and Balban had published their cases, but he did not refer to either of them in his article. The reason for this omission is understandable when one recalls that in the early nineteenth century, doctors did not have at their disposal massive indexes of the medical literature, such as *Index Medicus,* which can contain thousands of pages for any given year of the literature organized by subject, author, or journal. In the past several years, even *Index Medicus* has become nearly obsolete because of the rise of Internet-based indexes, such as Medline or PubMed. With a few keystrokes, for instance, to type in "cholera," a researcher will find hundreds if not thousands of articles listed. The computer will sort by author, date, or keyword. To delve into a more specific point, one can search for relevant articles on a disease that pertain only to diagnostics, or to therapeutics, or to the microbiology of the disease.

But in 1913, unless doctors happened to have read a previous article, they had little way to efficiently search the medical literature. This seemingly minor point—the lack of prior reference—was not without its consequences. Priority, as we will see, is very important in scientific nomenclature. In this case, the term that was used throughout Europe was ECM, even though Afzelius had reported his case of EM first.

In 1921 Afzelius published another article on this unusual erythema. This time, he reported on six personal cases, including the one in 1909 that was the substance of his earlier report and another case that he saw in 1908. In this report, Afzelius referred to the previous reports by Balban and Lipschutz, but he was unable to find other references in the literature. Afzelius regarded the clinical picture of EM to be pathognomonic, which is to say, the presence of the circular, red bull's-eye pattern of the rash by itself conclusively established the diagnosis. According to Harvard pathologist Dr. Gustav Dammin in 1989, Afzelius "considered EM to be an important lesion, since the recognition of it and knowledge of its natural course [to resolve spontaneously] would encourage use of conservative management and discourage attempts to modify its course." Dammin also notes that Afzelius titled his 1921 paper "Erythema Chronicum Migrans." The reason for this is not apparent because the narrative refers to ECM only four times, to EM nine times, and to the nonspecific "das Erythem" (the erythema) ten times.

As if not to be outdone, two years later, in 1923, Lipschutz again published on the rash, reviewing his own experience and that of others, including Afzelius. Lipschutz was able to catalogue a total of sixteen reported cases. He believed that the lesion began as a single red spot, often on the lower extremities, and noted that even though a red advancing edge would spread over a large area, the patient remained well, without fever or other symptoms. Although he did not include tick bite as an important feature, he did record that of the sixteen cases, five were preceded by a tick bite and another five, by some unspecified insect bite.

The European medical literature was even richer in terms of the breadth of manifestations associated with this unusual erythema. In 1922, Dr. Charles Garin (then an intern) and Dr. Bujadoux wrote a most interesting case report. In fact, this was another first-of-kind report in the medical literature. The patient was a thirty-eight-year-old sheep farmer who had been bitten by a sheep tick on his left buttock on June 14, 1922. Being a farmer with livestock and dogs, he was familiar with ticks and removed it without giving it a second thought. About three weeks later, he developed a painful illness of rapid onset that made him anxious because of its unusual nature. He consulted his local physician, who noticed that the man's pain was severe and followed the course of the sciatic nerve, on the same side as the tick bite. The other noteworthy finding was a large, tender ring of erythema, about the size of a five-franc coin. Furthermore, a lymph gland in the left groin was swollen.

The area of erythema enlarged and became uniformly red without any blisters. The rash grew to cover both of the man's buttocks and moved down the left leg to the knee and up onto the back and abdomen. But despite the striking nature of the rash, it was the pain that was so distinctive. Over the course of July and August, the man's pain spread to radiate down both sciatic nerves and then began to involve areas innervated by the intercostals nerves (the nerves between the ribs) as well. Finally, the pain became excruciating and even extended as far as the right brachial plexus in the shoulder and arm. Even morphine failed to provide the man with significant relief from the pain. Finally, on the advice of the local doctor, on September 16 the patient traveled to Lyon, where Dr. Garin immediately hospitalized him.

Drs. Garin and Bujadoux catalogued their findings. In general, they found the man to be anxious and "shivering," but he had no fever and his heart, lungs, and abdomen were normal. The sensation, reflexes, and pupils were normal. But they did find marked weakness of the right deltoid muscle with atrophy, or wasting, of the bulk of the muscle. The patient also had abnormal shoulder motion. Concerned that the patient could have a radiculitis (inflammation of the nerve roots that exit the spinal cord) or meningitis (inflammation of the membranes that cover the spinal cord and brain), Garin and Bujadoux performed a spinal tap on October 3.

The spinal cord exits the bottom of the brain like a string on a balloon. Years of evolution have ensured that the fragile brain and spinal cord are well protected by bone—the skull in the case of the brain, and the spine in the case of the spinal cord. The bony spinal column is an engineering and evolutionary marvel that simultaneously protects the cord while allowing the organism maximal flexibility and movement. Inside this bony sanctuary lie three additional layers of tissues, collectively called the *meninges*. Inside of these lies the cerebrospinal fluid—a kind of shock absorber—that further protects the brain and cord from the jabs and jolts of daily life.

Patients often become anxious when told they need a spinal tap, but in truth, it is a simple and straightforward procedure that has been performed since 1891. The purpose of the test is to get a sample of the normally crystal clear, colorless cerebrospinal fluid for analysis. Despite the plethora of high-tech, less invasive tests, such as the computed tomographic scan and magnetic resonance imaging, which allow doctors to "see" the farthest recesses of the brain and spinal cord without recourse to needle or scalpel, some situations remain for which there is no substitute for analyzing the spinal fluid directly.

The procedure is quite simple. With the back curved forward, as if the patient were in a fetal position, the bones of the spine open so that a doctor can pass a needle through openings in the bone, through the layers of the meninges, and into the cerebrospinal fluid. The spinal cord stops a few inches above where the doctor places the needle, so there is no danger of hitting the cord. Collectively, the bundle of nerve roots that float in this fluid-filled space look like a horse's tail, thus earning the name *cauda equina* from ancient anatomists. When nerve roots, or radicles, becomes inflamed, doctors diagnose radiculitis; they diagnose meningitis when the spinal fluid contains many cells or a high protein level.

In the case of Garin and Bujadoux's patient, the fluid was abnormal. The color was clear, but the protein level was elevated and white blood cells were present. No microorganisms were seen under the microscope. Thus, they diagnosed radiculitis with a mild meningitis. A test called the Wasserman reaction, a common test for syphilis at the time, was also weakly positive, so the patient was treated with four injections of neoarsphenamine, formerly used as an antisyphilitic agent, and three doses of mercury cyanide. He improved although motion in his right arm remained restricted. On October 17, the patient asked to be discharged. Given the treatments to which he was subjected, it is perhaps fortuitous that his request was granted. The patient continued to improve through October and November of 1922, but while the pain subsided, the arm limitations persisted.

Garin and Bujadoux reported this case as "a definite case of tick paralysis." On the other hand, they distinguished their case from others of tick paralysis by noting the unusual erythema and the fact that the species of tick involved was the *Ixodes* tick rather than the usual *Dermacentor*. It is of historical interest that they, like the group at Yale some fifty years later, became involved with their patient in the early autumn and recognized that any subsequent investigation would need to wait until the following spring. "We propose to collect ticks in the village where our patient lives next spring and to try to reproduce, consequent to their bites, the same illness in animals," they wrote. "The virus must then be looked for (in our inoculated animals) not in the blood but in the central nervous system, particularly in the anterior horn cells of the white matter and in the meninges, these being the organs affected in our patient." There is no record of this subsequent investigation.

Garin and Bujadoux did not connect the red rash with ECM, but the next European investigator who saw such a patient and recorded it did. The Swedish dermatologist Sven Hellerstrom reported a case in 1930 of a forty-nine-year-old mechanic with ECM and meningitis. This patient's skin eruption began on the lower trunk, and during the months the rash migrated, the patient developed chronic meningitis of unclear etiology. Hellerstrom speculated that the meningitis and erythema were related. He also emphatically made the point that because the reference by Afzelius predated that of Lipschutz, the correct terminology was ECM Afzelii, not Lipschutzi. This emphasis on the priority of Afzelius led to a dispute between Hellerstrom and Lipschutz—not the last disagreement regarding names in this saga, as we will see.

Hellerstrom's documentation and bibliography in that 1930 paper were fairly extensive at the time. Given the fact that Garin and Bujadoux had published in relatively obscure journals (although they republished their work in 1923 in *Lyon Medecine*), it is almost certain that Hellerstrom had been unaware of their contribution.

Nearly twenty years later, in November 1949, Hellerstrom presented his continued work on the subject of ECM in Cincinnati at a medical conference sponsored by the Southern Medical Association. His 1950 article in the *Southern Journal of Medicine* is the one that Dr. Scrimenti remembers and that led him to make the correct diagnosis, for the first time in North America, of ECM. In this article, Hellerstrom, now with two decades more experience in the area, made a number of conclusions. For one, he was convinced that the association between ECM and meningitis was more than just a coincidence because he had seen or read about several other cases, tallying at least six (not including the case from Lyon). Second, he was convinced that the disease was transmitted by tick bite (or occasionally perhaps by mosquito bite). "In the Stockholm area," he wrote, "cases of ECM are far from rare. Counting my private patients only, from 1935 to 1948 I have seen more than 30 instances of the condition. That the eruption is evoked by a tick bite is, in my opinion, a definitely established fact." He further noted that some patients had multiple areas of rash and wondered whether this was from multiple tick bites of which the patient was unaware, but he was not clear about the cause of this phenomenon. He also reasoned that given the high frequency of tick bites and the relatively low frequency of ECM, that most patients bitten do not contract ECM. He also documented that ECM, even when accompanied by meningitis, resolved spontaneously.

Hellerstrom made several other conclusions in the 1950 article that may seem both fantastic and prescient in light of subsequent history. He maintained that the disease was caused by a kind of bacterium called a spirochete. He also was certain that both the ECM and the meningitis were improved by penicillin therapy. At the same time, Hellerstrom thought that some of the manifestations were "allergic" and that "consequently, the condition belongs to the field of allergy." He recognized the conflict associated with these last two assertions. Why should an allergic disease improve with antibiotics?

8 • Further Work in Europe

Hellerstrom had good, if indirect, reasons for believing that the responsible organism was a spirochete. One of those reasons had to do with a doctor working with him at the Karolinska Institute in Sweden—Carl Lennhoff. Lennhoff had trained in dermatology in Breslau and Hamburg, Germany, and was the head of the Dermatology Department in Magdeburg when, in 1933, he was forced to flee the Nazi regime. In Sweden, he ultimately continued his work, which involved developing special stains to examine spirochetes under the microscope.

Spirochetes are one of the countless microorganisms, or "bugs" as physicians frequently call them, with which humans share this planet Earth. Life has evolved along multiple pathways, and microorganisms that cause human infection are of various classes, each of which has found some measure of success in the evolutionary process. From the human perspective, it is easy to lose sight of the fact that each of these classes of organisms—which include bacteria, viruses, fungi, parasites, and possibly new ones called prions—has evolved over tens of thousands of years into its own niche. Furthermore, bacteria have evolved into several subgroups.

Viruses are tiny organisms that cause diseases such as the common cold, hepatitis, measles, yellow fever, and chickenpox. Some viruses, for example the influenza virus, can be deadly; the strain responsible for the 1918 flu pandemic killed more than forty million people worldwide. More recently, the human immunodeficiency virus (HIV) that causes AIDS is another vicious player on the stage of microorganisms. Viruses are much smaller than bacteria and have evaded detection by medical scientists for a much longer time. Nor did they respond to early antibiotics. Recently, however, with breakthroughs in molecular biology and virology, scientists have found antimicrobials that will attack and kill viruses, too.

Next are the fungi, such as histoplasma and cryptococcus. These organisms are ubiquitous in nature and will attack humans here and there, when the opportunity is right. Some fungi cause life-threatening diseases whereas others cause relatively harmless conditions such as ringworm and athlete's foot.

Another group of bugs are the parasites—worms and protozoa—which cause some of the most common maladies on the planet, from pinworm to malaria. Malaria, caused by a single-cell protozoan that infects red blood cells, produces spiking fevers and shaking chills in those affected. Although rare in the United States, it is probably the most common infectious disease in the world, infecting more than three hundred million people each year and killing several million of them. Another much less common protozoan disease is called babesiosis, which will later play a role in our story.

The word *prion,* for "proteinaceous infectious agent," was coined in 1982 by a neurologist who believed these new agents to be responsible for several neurodegenerative diseases that resemble those caused by slow viruses.

Some of the group of bugs known as bacteria have specialized under evolutionary pressure into subgroups, including rickettsia, mycobacteria, and spirochetes. The well-known bacteria staphylococcus and streptococcus cause skin infections; the pneumococcus bacterium causes pneumonia, which has killed countless millions worldwide; the bubonic plague bacterium wiped out a good percentage of

Europe during the Middle Ages; and *E. coli* causes many simple urinary tract infections and some diarrheal illnesses.

The rickettsial agents, like viruses, must live inside cells. The agent that causes Rocky Mountain spotted fever is a rickettsia, as is the agent of epidemic typhus. The most notorious mycobacterium causes tuberculosis, the most common cause of death in the United States in the year 1900. Another mycobacterium has emerged as a serious problem in HIV-infected patients. Still another can cause a chronic skin infection that one can get from merely cleaning out a home aquarium.

Of the group of bugs called spirochetes, so named because of their unique spiral-shaped or corkscrew appearance under the microscope, the most well-known is *Treponema pallidum,* the agent of the venereal disease syphilis. This infection is spread via sexual contact and primarily affects the skin, heart, and nervous system. Syphilis was very common in the mid-twentieth century, and could be deadly, so scientists tried to culture the spirochete. Microbiologists can easily culture staphylococci or streptococci and even the plague bacillus. But *Treponema pallidum* was different; it could not be cultured (a situation that still persists). With the proper stains and the right equipment, however, it, and other spirochetes, could be seen under a microscope—which is what Carl Lennhoff was trying to do.

But first, some background. The *Treponemes* represent one genus within the family of spirochetes. The words *genus* and *family,* as used here, are part of the way that humans have tried to impose a structure on the complicated world around us—by naming things. Our current system dates back about 250 years, when the Swedish naturalist Carolus Linnaeus tried to help create order out of a rather chaotic classification system that was a mosaic of various systems that had been developed over centuries.

Linnaeus grouped all living creatures into two kingdoms—plant or animal, although since Linnaeus the number of kingdoms has grown to account for organisms such as bacteria and single-celled organisms. From the kingdom flows a cascade of progressively smaller and more connected groupings: phylum, class, order, family, genus, and species. The last two, the genus and the species, are the italicized Latin words that one sees in the scientific name of something, such as *Treponema* (the genus) *pallidum* (the species). The genus is a noun, and the species an adjective, which often describes the location where the organism is found or the name of a person who discovered it.

While this may seem like much ado about nothing, anyone who has gone beyond the intermediate level of learning a foreign language can sympathize with Linnaeus's desire for a common nomenclature. Initially, one is proud of oneself for knowing the word for *bird, tree,* or *flower.* But rapidly, this is not enough, and in the case of birds, for instance, one needs to distinguish among finches, swallows, and seagulls. A bilingual bird lover would then need to learn the names of the various types of swallows. In order for biologists to speak with each other, they needed a common language.

So the "organizational chart" for the spirochete *Treponema pallidum* would look like this:

- Kingdom: Prokaryotae
- Phylum: Gracilicutes
- Class: Scotobacteria
- Order: Spirochaetales
- Family: Spirochaetaceae
- Genus: Treponema
- Species: pallidum

As biologists unlock more and more of the genetic secrets of these bugs and are able to sequence genes and decode proteins, reclassifications and subclassifications are becoming increasingly common, as is the concept of different "strains," but for now, we will focus on genus and species.

When Carl Lennhoff escaped Nazi Germany and went to Sweden, he was working with spirochetes. Unfortunately, he lost some of his work in his hasty departure. In a treatise on his work that he published in 1948, he wrote, "The investigations, on which I am going to report, date in part as far back as 20–25 years. I was obliged to abandon my notes pertaining to this work when fleeing . . . and they must be considered lost. Thus I must ask you to be indulgent if I cannot make definite statements on some points."

Lennhoff, according to Nils Thyresson, a dermatologist active at the Karolinska Institute at the same time as Lennhoff, "was obsessed by the idea that he would be able to visualize spirochetes in a lot of skin diseases with hitherto unknown etiology. One of those diseases was erythema migrans." For bacteria to be seen on a slide under a microscope, stains must be applied to the tissue or bacteria. The tissues and bacteria absorb these colorful stains differently. One of the most commonly applied stains in bacteriology, Gram's stain, forms the basis for dividing various bacteria into two major groups. Based on the composition of their outer cell membrane, most major bacteria either take up the stain (they are Gram-positive) or they don't (they are Gram-negative). This is not merely a chromatic curiosity but forms the basis for how doctors select antibiotic therapy.

It turns out that spirochetes could not be visualized with Gram's stain, so Lennhoff had to devise a different staining method. In 1948, he used a combination of mercury chloride, which interacted with the spirochetes, and ammonium sulfide. The resultant mercury sulfide was visible and Lennhoff was able to see spirochetes. But there was a serious problem. He began finding spirochetes almost everywhere he looked. He found them in patients with psoriasis and eczema; with German measles, chickenpox, rashes resulting from infections on the heart valves, and numerous other skin conditions; and, relevant to this story, with ECM. Needless to say, this caused great excitement in the field of dermatology because of the prospect of finding a cause for so many diseases whose etiologies remained obscure in 1950.

Unfortunately, Lennhoff's work was later shown to be erroneous. But his work nonetheless raised interest in and awareness of spirochetes, and before he died, he donated money to the Karolinska Institute for spirochetal research. In 1950, however, his findings were still thought to be accurate, helping support Hellerstrom's opinion that ECM was caused by a spirochete. Another reason was the fact that drugs known to help spirochetal infections made ECM vanish far faster than it would do so spontaneously. One of these was penicillin.

In 1950 penicillin had only recently been introduced generally. Alexander Fleming's report of his discovery in 1929 of the miraculous mold that killed bacteria had lain unrecognized in the medical literature for ten years until Howard Florey and Ernst Chain at Oxford University resurrected the idea and performed numerous tests in the laboratory on bacteria. Next they successfully tested it on animals. When they published their results in 1940, the knowledge of penicillin's effect on bacteria had reached the average physician, and its use arrived at the bedside. However, this happened during the Second World War, so much of the drug that was produced went toward the war effort, delaying the general availability of penicillin by several years. But within about five years of the end of the war, it was tested on ECM. Then in 1955, German physician Erich Binder and colleagues reported on their experiments with ECM and penicillin. Procedurally, these men followed in the footsteps of another German scientist, as well as other doctors around the world.

The advancement of medical science has been punctuated now and again with self-experimentation. Dr. Max Von Pettenkofer, for instance, when he was developing his theories about the pathogenesis of cholera, did more than put his money where his mouth was—he put the *bacteria* in his mouth to conclusively try to prove his theory that cholera was not transmissible person to person. On October 7, 1892, he swallowed a large dose of the bacteria derived from a patient who had died of the disease. In order to preempt the argument that his stomach acid would kill the cholera bacillus, he drank some bicarbonate of sodium to neutralize the acidity. He fell ill with abdominal cramps and diarrhea, but improved after a week. Although many critics at the time argued that the experiment proved little, Pettenkofer pronounced it a complete success. (In fact, Pettenkofer had suffered a mild, naturally acquired cholera attack in the past from which he had recovered and which may have left him with partial immunity.)

Another, and perhaps more tragic, instance of self-experimentation occurred in the battle against yellow fever. In 1900 Dr. Walter Reed was director of a commission charged with investigating the cause and transmission of yellow fever in Cuba. The leading theories of the day were that the disease was spread by inanimate objects (such as bedsheets and clothing), that is was spread person-to-person, and that mosquitoes were involved in the transmission. While Reed was in Washington, D.C., other members of the commission conducted experiments on themselves with mosquito bites. One man nearly died, and one did die, making the ultimate "sacrifice" to higher ideals that Pettenkofer had earlier identified: "I would have died in the service of science like a soldier on the field of honor. Health and life are, as I have so often said, very great earthly goods but not the highest for man. Man, if he will rise above the animals, must sacrifice both life and health for the higher ideals."

In 1955, Binder and his colleagues embarked upon this same path and performed an experiment on themselves. Fortunately, they were experimenting with a disease that was not fatal and that could be treated. These doctors took tissue samples from the outer ring of erythema of patients with active ECM and transplanted the biopsy specimen into themselves. All three men developed ECM in the ensuing weeks. They extended their findings by taking a specimen from one of them and transplanting it yet again into another volunteer who also developed the rash. Then they treated all of the recipients with penicillin, and the rash disappeared in every case within a few days.

Thus, twenty years before the outbreak of arthritis and EM in coastal Connecticut, European doctors were convinced that an infectious agent caused ECM. Nobody had successfully isolated that organism, but the consensus was that it was almost certainly a bacterium, and possibly a spirochete. They further concluded, partly on the basis of empirical therapeutic trials and partly on the basis of the data from Binder and colleagues, that whatever its cause, ECM could be treated with penicillin.

But two other threads were woven into the fabric of this understanding of ECM. The first dates to 1883 when the German physician Alfred Buchwald described a thirty-six-year-old man who suffered for sixteen years with what he termed "diffuse idiopathic skin atrophy." The man's entire left thigh to the knee was involved. As the name that Buchwald gave the condition implies, he knew of no cause. The skin became so thin that it was described as having the appearance of "crumpled cigarette paper." Over the ensuing decades, other European physicians reported similar cases, and in 1902, Karl Herxheimer and Kuno Hartmann described a number of these other cases and applied the name acrodermatitis chronica atrophicans, or ACA. This descriptive name means that the condition tended to affect the extremities *(acro)* and was typified by a chronic thinning *(chronica atrophicans)* of the skin. By evaluating more cases, Herxheimer and Hartmann were able to distinguish an earlier inflammatory phase of the disease and a later atrophic one.

This disease had been described in the United States but almost always in European immigrants. In a group of forty-five such patients reported from North America in 1945, seven of them had arthritis or arthralgia (pain in the joints without objective swelling) although the authors of this report did not believe that the joint problems were related to the skin problem.

The other thread that was gradually woven into the fabric of understanding began in 1911 when the Swiss physician Jean Louis Burckhardt described a sixty-year-old woman with a one-by-three-inch red plaque (a flat raised area on the skin) on her upper arm. When he examined the tissue under the microscope, it had the appearance of a lymph node. Other physicians began to report the same phenomenon, and in 1929, Mulzer and Keining made an association between ACA and this odd lymph tissue, which they termed lymphocytoma.

In 1943, Swedish dermatologist Bo Bafverstedt published a monograph on the subject of lymphocytoma that continued to see links, noting that in his work with forty-one patients, ECM had been present in four and ACA in three others.

Besides these three threads of ACA, lymphocytoma, and ECM in the fabric of understanding the skin findings, meningitis comes back into the picture with the work of Alfred Bannwarth in the 1940s. By 1944, Bannwarth had reported on twenty-six patients with chronic lymphocytic meningitis but failed to make any connection with the work in 1922 of Garin and Bujadoux. Just as the patient of these previous doctors has suffered radiculitis, or severe pain along the nerve roots, so, too, did many of Bannwarth's patients. Furthermore, some of them had other problems with facial nerve paralysis and other disorders of the so-called "cranial nerves," or the nerves that exit via the base of the brain.

Thus, on the eve of the introduction of penicillin to the medical community after the Second World War, a loose connection had been made between three rashes—ECM, ACA, and lymphocytoma. Some investigators also noted an association between some of these and chronic lymphocytic meningitis.

And the use of antibiotics to treat the three skin diseases also continued to show promise. In 1949, Nils Thyresson of the Karolinska Institute reported on the use of penicillin in fifty-seven patients with ACA. Seven were cured and twenty-eight showed major improvement. Other antibiotics were also used, and tetracycline seemed to have some activity in treating this disease. Nobody knew what the causative organism was, but these findings stimulated the search.

In 1950, G. E. Bianchi noted a positive effect from penicillin in patients with lymphocytoma. Antibiotic therapy also proved efficacious in 1954, when Hans Gotz and colleagues from the Department of Dermatology at the University of Munich in Germany performed the first successful transmission experiments on ACA. Gotz and his coinvestigators took skin biopsy specimens from patients with ACA and transplanted the tissue into their own skin. They began feeling pain in the joints and an altered sensitivity in the skin and developed a red rash with characteristics of ECM and ACA. All of these changes disappeared with antibiotic therapy.

Also in 1954, Jean-Marie Paschoud, from Lausanne, Switzerland, noted an association among lymphocytoma, tick bite, and the meningoradiculitis that Garin and Bujadoux had reported—a connection that Bannwarth had missed. Paschoud also noted the association between ECM and lymphocytoma, leading him to repeat the transmission experiments that Gotz and Binder had done with ACA and ECM, respectively. The Swiss investigator used material from patients with lymphocytoma. His experiments were also successful in transmitting the rash from person to person.

Therefore, by the late 1950s, experiments had established that some unknown agent was present in the skin of patients with all three of these conditions—ECM, ACA, and lymphocytoma—and that this agent could be transmitted from one human to another by transplanting affected skin into the recipient. According to Dr. Klaus Weber, a German dermatologist who catalogued all of these contributions from the European literature, "all of these experiences together left no doubt to dermatologists in Europe that antibiotic treatment was indicated for these conditions; this was standard practice!"

9 • The Blind Men and the Elephant

"Standard practice" in the United States was not yet clear, however, especially considering that doctors on this side of the Atlantic had not yet made several "connections" that were perhaps known in Europe. Furthermore, the backgrounds and experiences of the group of rheumatologists at Yale and the two doctors at the Submarine Medical Center in Groton varied considerably. How they responded to this new illness and the questions of how to treat it can be interpreted in the context of the story of the blind men and the elephant.

The origin of this well-known tale is unknown. Most believe it to be a Hindu folktale from India, whereas others contend that it began in China with the Han Dynasty (206 B.C. to A.D. 220). There is also an African version. Some versions include four blind men, others six. Whatever the details, the story goes something like this. Six blind men encounter an elephant for the first time and seek to discover more about the nature of this unknown creature. The first touches the elephant's wide, firm side and claims that the elephant is like a wall. The second touches the round and twisting trunk and believes the pachyderm to be like a snake. The third feels the smooth, sharp tusk and pronounces that the elephant is most like a spear. The fourth man reaches for the animal's broad and floppy ear and concludes that the elephant is like a fan. The fifth, who gropes for the leg, believes that the elephant is like a tree trunk. The last blind man grabs the tail and says that the elephant is like a rope.

In some versions, a "truly" wise man, such as the Rajah of the palace in one account or an older, worldier blind man in another, is able to put the puzzle in perspective. Some people interpret this story in a religious context, claiming that knowing the elephant is like knowing God, different for different individuals. Others have a more secular interpretation, understanding the story as showing that cultural biases distort how we experience the truth. Each of the blind men was partially right, but none grasped the entire truth, in part because of his limited perspective of the reality in question and in part because of his individual cultural perspective.

In the case of the physicians from the submarine base, Dr. William Mast was an internist, and Dr. William Burrows was a dermatologist. Their reality included four patients with an acute skin rash that was large, red, and inflamed. Some of the patients had fevers and chills and other symptoms of acute disease. To these two doctors, even before they learned of the European experience, it made perfect sense that the condition might improve with antibiotics. Then, as each patient seemed to improve with antibiotics, their direct experience with their patients validated their notion. Later, they became aware of the European literature that demonstrated that this rash was ECM and could be cured by antibiotics. Their bias was that an antibiotic-sensitive agent, likely a bacterium, spread the infection.

Simultaneously, the group at Yale was based in the Rheumatology Division, so these doctors understandably focused on the joint manifestations of the malady. From their point of view, there was far less evidence that this was an acute process that would respond to antibiotics; in fact, their reality suggested that it was entirely self-limited. By the time they saw their patients, the rash had long since disappeared, in many cases without antibiotic treatment. Even by the summer of 1976, when they began to see patients with the rash, it seemed to disappear rapidly in some patients who were not treated with antibiotics and lasted for a longer time in others who did receive antibiotics. Even the arthritis resolved without antibiotics, a seemingly minor fact that continued to fascinate Dr. Malawista.

In their initial report in the January 1977 issue of *Arthritis and Rheumatism,* the Yale group called the disease *Lyme arthritis.* This made perfect sense to them because, after all, this was an outbreak of arthritis centered in the town of Lyme. Naming a disease after the place in which it is first described is commonplace. In this initial report on Lyme arthritis, the Yale group wrote: "The best treatment for this illness is not clear. Some physicians [they refer to the European literature] have reported that penicillin or tetracycline results in disappearance of the skin lesions but others have found antibiotics ineffective. Four of the patients with expanding skin lesions received penicillin but still developed arthritis."

In their next clinical publication in the June 1977 issue of *Annals of Internal Medicine,* Steere and colleagues noted that many doctors had reported on the utility of antibiotics for both the neurological and the skin conditions (they catalogued twelve reports) but pointed out that others (one report) disagreed. "We remain skeptical," they wrote, "that antibiotic therapy helps; the large variation in the natural course of the disease makes it difficult to evaluate whether the observed improvement in the individual patient would have occurred anyway. Eight of our patients received penicillin, erythromycin, or cephalexin before entering the study because of the skin lesion. In one of them, the lesion persisted despite therapy, longer than in any of the other study patients, and seven of the eight still developed joint, neurologic, or cardiac abnormalities."

With the benefit of hindsight, we know that some of the antibiotics, such as cephalexin, and some of the doses prescribed or durations of treatment were ineffective. But at the time, none of this was clear.

Perhaps this was simply a case of seeing what one wants to see. But scientists are not immune from contextual and cultural biases. In this case, the context was a chronic, late manifestation of a disease versus an acute, early one. And the culture was that of a rheumatologist versus that of a dermatologist.

Steere remembers this period well. Besides the fact that some of the antibiotic-treated patients had persistent or worsened symptoms, he had several lines of evidence and good reasons for believing that the pathogen was a virus and not a bacterium. For one, he had examined many biopsy specimens of synovial tissue. "Viruses are hard to find," says Steere, "whereas bacteria are large and should be sitting there in the synovial tissue. We thought we'd have seen a bacterium in the tissue, if that's what it was."

The second line of evidence was the rash. Of the first fifty-seven patients studied, thirteen of them recalled an unusual rash but forty-four did not. And even of the ones who described a rash, "they didn't all describe it the same way," Steere remembers. "So it wasn't that you had thirteen people who described the same thing. And you could always wonder that within a community, maybe thirteen people would have an insect bite in the summer. But some of them described it in a really dramatic way, and so I remember thinking, What is this that these people are describing? Has anyone ever heard of something like that? And so it was a matter of talking to people. I spoke to the dermatologists at Yale and said, 'Have you ever seen anything like this?' I had drawn pictures of what had been described to me. One of them said that there had been a conference in dermatology earlier in the year by two physicians from the submarine base and they had presented several cases that had unusual skin lesions. He wondered if it was the same thing."

Steere's conversation with his colleagues established that the Navy doctors believed the rash was ECM, which had been described in Europe. Steere looked up the condition in a standard dermatology reference. "It was a small section [in the book]," he recalls, which noted that the rash occurred at the site of a tick bite and that there was some indication that neurological phenomena also occurred in some patients. Steere remembers that usually, "it was self-limited, though there were some people who thought it could be treated with penicillin." Steere called Burrows and they compared their experiences. The Navy doctors cooperated by referring some of their patients to be studied at Yale. Some of those patients who were treated with antibiotics later developed arthritis. So Steere and Malawista were still convinced that a virus caused the disease, and this was the official stance of the Yale group in 1976.

That summer was an exciting time for them. It was the first summer that they could study the disease and learn more about it as well as *see* some of the rashes that previously they had only heard about. When they encountered patients with the rash, they biopsied it so that they could look at it under the microscope, where they saw the same nonspecific changes that Mast and Burrows had seen. Doctors also learned that most people did not recall a particular insect bite that occurred at the site where the rash developed.

Other pieces to the puzzle began to appear as well. During that summer of 1976, the Yale group asked physicians in the affected towns to identify and refer patients who either had recent onset of the ECM rash or Lyme arthritis. Because they were now seeing patients from the very start of their symptoms, the Yale doctors were able to evaluate patients prospectively (that is, examine them during the acute phase of the illness at the time it was occurring). Steere, still a junior fellow at Yale, took the lead and personally evaluated all of these patients. He tested blood samples for literally hundreds of microorganisms. When he found fluid in a joint, he analyzed it. He biopsied rashes and synovial tissue and examined the tissue microscopically.

For all of the reports that had emerged over nearly one hundred years from Europe, this was the first concentrated and extensive epidemiological effort brought to bear on this phenomenon. The effort was massive, prospective, and deliberate and was being accomplished by a university with world-class resources. The power of epidemiological analysis became clear, and the Yale investigators made several extremely important observations. The onset of symptoms of those patients presenting with rash occurred earlier in the season than those who presented with arthritis. Thus, it became clear that the disease occurred in stages—first the skin, later the joints. Furthermore, although there had been an occasional coincidence of arthritis and

ECM, the association of arthritis and rash had never been clearly established in the European literature. Another observation the Yale group made was that not infrequently, patients had multiple ECM lesions. This finding had been reported in Sweden in 1965 but had not been thought to occur commonly in Europe.

During that summer of 1976, the Yale investigators also began to observe other manifestations of Lyme arthritis. "It became apparent that it was a multisystem disease," Steere says. "When we prospectively followed the patients with the skin lesion, more than half developed arthritis. And then also some developed meningitis or Bell's palsy, which we did not expect. And then some people developed carditis [an inflammation of the heart muscle], which we also didn't expect." The meningitis was of the lymphocytic (nonbacterial) type—recalling the findings of Garin and Bujadoux in 1922 and Bannwarth in 1941. This link provided an additional reason that the Yale group did not think that antibiotics were indicated. The Europeans believed Bannwarth's syndrome to be due to a virus and did not use antibiotics to treat it.

Two patients developed heart arrhythmias, and one of them, complete heart block, in which the heart's electrical system fails to conduct the impulse from the upper chambers to the lower ones, leading to a dangerously slow heart rate. This was a new finding and helped evolve the thinking about the disease. When someone had the joint manifestation, it was referred to as Lyme arthritis, as opposed to rheumatoid or gouty arthritis. But when a patient presented with rash and a paralyzed facial nerve, or fever and an irregular heartbeat, it no longer made sense to call it Lyme arthritis. And so the term *Lyme disease* was soon born.

Despite these important advances, the cause of the disease, whether a virus, a bacterium, or another organism, continued to remain unknown. In a letter from Steere and Malawista to the patients in the study dated May 18, 1976, the doctors summarized the findings of the investigation. Of the joint problems, they wrote: "We would like to re-emphasize that we believe 'Lyme arthritis' to be a relatively mild type of arthritis which may be self-limited. We can hope that patients will have no permanent difficulty from it."

As one can imagine, the local population was concerned about this new disease, especially given that many affected individuals were children, whose joints were terribly swollen. Like Legionnaire's disease the summer before and toxic shock syndrome before that, Lyme arthritis was attracting a great deal of notoriety and media attention. Articles began to appear in the local and national press. Some coverage fueled these concerns.

Reporting for the *New York Times* on July 18, 1976, Boyce Rensberger wrote an article whose page-one headline announced "A new type of arthritis found in Lyme." The article chronicled the details of the epidemiological investigation, but it began on a rather sensational note: "A teenage boy suddenly developed severe pains in his leg and could not walk. His attacks lasting a week or more, have come and gone several times. Just a few miles away, a 9-year-old girl woke up to find her knee swollen to twice its normal size. She spent weeks in a wheelchair. Down the street from her, another child was stricken with painful swollen joints that left him crippled for weeks. . . . People began to fear something more than a coincidence was at work."

Nine days later, on July 27, local political representatives organized a town meeting in the Lyme high school auditorium. Steere and Malawista presented their findings. Approximately 350 people came to listen, some from as far away as Norwalk, Connecticut, and Pawtucket and Providence, Rhode Island. By then, the news was spreading, and some people reported to have known people who might have the new disease.

According to articles in local papers, such as the *New London Day* (July 28) and the *Old Lyme Gazette* (July 29), the medical researchers and local public health officials tended to downplay the seriousness of the disease. But some in the audience told other stories. One woman from Norwalk said she had been bedridden and incapacitated from November 1975 though May 1976 with swollen joints, which she believed to have been due to Lyme arthritis. Concerns were expressed that Lyme would be considered "Arthritis City" and that people would stop sending their children to summer camps in the area or renting vacation cottages. State Health Commissioner Douglas

S. Lloyd tried to assure people that there was presently no reason to label the disease a widespread danger, although he did say that the disease "appears to be a generalized phenomena [sic] in the area."

National news magazines picked up the story and so, too, did some of the tabloids. One, The Star, ran a story titled "Mystery Illness Cripples Victims in Three Towns."

Another controversy that was aired at the town meeting was the effectiveness of antibiotics in treating the malady. At this point, the Yale group still maintained that antibiotics were of no value and that symptomatic treatment with aspirin and drainage of affected swollen joints was appropriate. But the Navy doctors, Mast and Burrows, whose experience by their second summer of dealing with ECM now included ten patients, felt stronger than ever that antibiotics clearly helped. In the Gazette article, Mast acknowledged that it was possible that the improvement of the rash with antibiotic therapy could have been coincidental; nevertheless, he and Burrows strongly believed that antibiotics should be prescribed.

When separately interviewed nearly twenty years after this town meeting, both Mast and Burrows independently recalled feeling that their opinions were being dismissed, in part because they were "Navy doctors." Recalls Mast: "Allen [Steere] at that time was very adamant about antibiotics having absolutely no role in the disease. We left with some feelings of animosity at that point. And the academic people made us feel like we obviously didn't know what we were doing. And we knew from our observations that we did."

Nevertheless, the Navy doctors tried to remain open-minded. They contacted their ten patients again and found that one of them had developed arthritis, "but we still had a 90 percent cure rate," remembers Burrows. And despite their different points of view about treatment, the two groups collaborated to some extent.

In a letter to the editor published in JAMA in November 1976, Mast and Burrows wrote: "On exchange of patients and information with Dr. Steere and the group at Yale investigating 'Lyme arthritis,' it is the consensus that we are dealing with the same process. It is apparent that the term 'Lyme arthritis' is much too restrictive, since there have been cases from the Connecticut and Rhode Island shores and the incidence is expected to be more widespread." An accompanying letter to the editor from two physicians from Hyannis, Massachusetts, described two additional cases that presented with rash but later developed arthritis. (The report does not state whether those patients were treated with antibiotics.)

Regarding treatment, the Yale group's opinion can be summarized in their letter of May 18, 1976, to the study patients: "The best treatment for the usually mild symptoms of arthritis is not yet clear. At present, we suggest taking only aspirin during symptomatic periods. In a few patients, knee swelling has persisted for months. Should this occur, we believe that continuing care by a physician is important."

10 • The Connection with Ticks

In that same letter to their patients, the Yale doctors asked for the patients' help, "by saving insects (particularly ticks) that bite you and your family." Since the earliest days of the investigation, this suspicion of an insect vector, likely a tick, had existed and stemmed from several lines of evidence.

Both Mrs. Mensch and Mrs. Murray had wondered about this possibility, sensing that the number of ticks in the area had exploded over the prior decade. When Dr. Steere first visited the Mensches, Mrs. Mensch mentioned that they had noticed an increase in the number of ticks over the past few years. Polly Murray notes in her book, *The Widening Circle*, that she frequently pulled ticks off family members and suspected that some of their symptoms were related to these bites. That was as far back as 1965. By 1973, she documents that she and her friends and neighbors began to notice an increase in the local tick population. Then there was the European data, which strongly suggested an association of the rash ECM and the bite of the tick *Ixodes ricinus*. Furthermore, the epidemiological data that Steere and his colleagues had assembled—the tight geographical clustering (areas outside of the town centers) and the temporal clustering (during the warm months of the year)—strongly suggested an insect vector. In 1976, when the Yale group saw the first patients with rash, they biopsied the skin lesions, and the appearance under the microscope was consistent with an arthropod bite.

Most patients did not remember being bitten by a tick, but some did, and during the summer of 1976, several patients with the rash brought the offending ticks to the doctors. One of them, Joe Dowhan, was a biologist with the Department of Environmental Protection for the State of Connecticut. "We were in Bluff Point, Connecticut," he recalls, "which is about two towns to the east of Lyme. It was early in the morning in early June, in a very heavily wooded area. And I had a lot of biological sampling gear, everything from collecting jars and nets to binoculars. . . . all of a sudden I felt a pinch on my neck and grabbed and pulled it off me and there was this tiny tick. I mean, it was strange; it really hurt. It was an instantaneous bite there. I flicked it off; it was a real tiny one. . . . after a few minutes, I got another bite on my knee. Again, it was a sharp pinch. I looked down and there it was, a tiny tick again. I was puzzled because I had been around ticks a lot as a field biologist my entire professional career. I had pulled thousands of ticks off me, and I had never had any bite me so aggressively, so instantaneously. I had a collecting jar with me. And so I took this little tick, it looked like a nymph, and threw it in the jar and proceeded."

Three days later, Dowhan developed a red rash in the area of one of the tick bites. He had seen the news reports and recalled an article in a magazine describing the Yale effort. He recalls reading that "some of the patients reported having a rash. They didn't know the cause but they were investigating the possibility that this may have been an arthropod-borne disease. Well, as the rashes grew, it didn't take a rocket scientist to know what I was coming down with. So around four or five days after I was bit, I called Dr. Steere.

"He spoke to me and examined me and then brought in a few interns or residents and he said, 'I think you have one of the earliest cases, but I'm pretty sure that's what you have, and would you be a

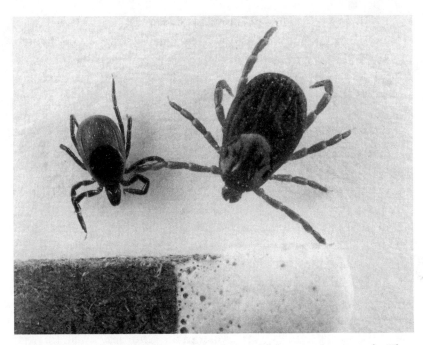

Figure 10. Two ticks seen in comparison with a common match. The larger tick is *Dermacentor variabilis* (the "dog tick," responsible for transmitting Rocky Mountain spotted fever) and the smaller is an adult *Ixodes scapularis* (the "deer tick," responsible for transmitting Lyme disease). (Photo by Darlyne Murawski.)

study patient of mine?' Ever the biologist, with a fascination in human biology as well, I said 'yes.' Then I said, 'and this is what gave it to me,' and I pulled out that jar with the tick. And of course everyone's eyebrows went up. And the folks from the School of Epidemiology came over and examined it. And the rest is history." The tick was identified as *Ixodes scapularis*, popularly known as the deer tick and related to its European cousin, *Ixodes ricinus*, which had been implicated as the vector for ECM in Europe (Figure 10).

Ticks have been around since antiquity. In an article published in *Nature* in 1965, British zoologist Don Arthur suggests that ticks may have been around since some of the earliest Egyptian dynasties. He notes that a tomb in Western Thebes, dating from approximately 1500 B.C., shows a hyenalike animal that has a distinctly ticklike parasite on it. More than a millennium later, in 355 B.C., the Greek philosopher and natural scientist Aristotle wrote in his *Historia animalium* that "ticks are generated from crouch grass." The notion that ticks spontaneously generate was wrong, of course, but Aristotle continues to note that "the ass has no lice or ticks, oxen have both . . . among dogs [ticks] are plentiful."

In A.D. 77, Pliny the Elder wrote of "the foulest and nastiest creatures that be—ill-favored ticks, an animal living on blood with its head always fixed and swelling, being one of the animals which has no exit [anus] for its food, it bursts with ever repletion and dies from actual nourishment." He also catalogues which animals have the most and the least number of ticks. The concept that ticks lack a terminal end to their alimentary, or gastrointestinal, tract is untrue, but the perception that ticks live on blood is correct.

Ticks have lived in North America for centuries as well. In 1754, Pehr Kalm, referring to ticks in land that is now the United States, is quoted as saying, "This small vile creature may, in the future, cause the inhabitants of this land great damage unless a method is discovered which will prevent it from increasing at such a shocking rate."

Biologists like to categorize and classify things. In part, this is simply the nature of biologists, but to be fair, the issue of nomenclature imparts issues of priority (as seen with the name for the rash ECM) and also helps scientists better understand both the history of a species and its relationships to other living things. This latter idea sometimes helps to shape our theories about the relationship of creatures to disease.

Strictly speaking, ticks are not insects. In the grand scheme of beasts both large and small, ticks belong to the phylum Arthropoda, and following the classification system begun by Linnaeus discussed in Chapter 8, their "organization chart" would look like this:

- Phylum: Arthropoda
- Class: Arachnida
- Order: Acarina
- Family: Ixodidae—"hard" ticks
                Argasidae—"soft" ticks
                Nuttalliellidae

The Nuttalliellidae contain no ticks that are of medical interest. The other two, however, play important roles in our story. The Ixodidae are known as "hard" ticks because of their hard exterior shield, which covers a portion of the dorsal surface. The Argasidae are referred to as "soft" ticks because of their soft, leatherlike outer skin.

The families are further subdivided into genera. In our story, the genera of hard ticks that play important roles are the *Ixodes, Dermacentor,* and *Amblyomma.* Of the soft ticks, the genus *Ornithodoros* will also play an important, if supporting, role. Within each of these genera, are species—about eight hundred in these two families. Within the *Ixodes* genus, we have already met the species *Ixodes ricinus* and *Ixodes scapularis.* (The genus name is often abbreviated, as in *I. ricinus* and *I. scapularis.*)

Ticks are obligate blood-sucking parasites, which means that they must find a blood meal from a vertebrate in order to change into their next stage of existence—no blood, no survival. Eggs released by adult female ticks hatch into larvae. These tiny, six-legged larvae must find a blood meal in order to molt into the next stage—a nymph. The nymph in turn must also find a blood meal to complete the cycle and change into an adult (Figure 11).

As a group, ticks are not very finicky in their feeding habits; nearly any vertebrate will do. However, particular species of ticks have their favorites. Another difference between the hard and soft ticks is that hard ticks usually feed on the vertebrate for several days whereas soft ticks obtain their blood meal in minutes or hours. But no matter how long it takes, during this blood meal, a tick infected by an infectious agent could transmit that agent to the vertebrate from which it feeds—whether it be human or animal.

One of the most successful chapters in American biology—the

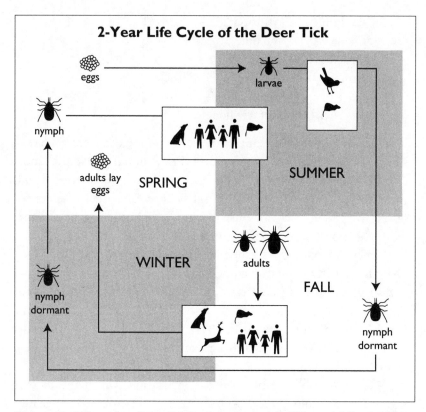

Figure 11. Life cycle of the *Ixodes scapularis* tick ("deer tick"), the tick found to transmit Lyme disease in the northeastern United States. (Courtesy of the American Lyme Disease Foundation, Somers, N.Y.)

discovery of the nature of Texas cattle fever—was an example of the latter. Dr. Theobald Smith, after graduating from Albany Medical College, landed a job with the Bureau of Animal Industry in Washington, D.C. In the late nineteenth century, as now, economic interests often drove research. In this case, cattle ranchers had noticed a problem with their cattle since the late 1860s, and Smith was assigned to solve it.

Southern ranchers would purchase healthy northern cattle, which they would graze with healthy southern cattle. All would be well until about a month later (and only in the summer months), when the northern cattle would begin to die en masse. Similarly, when southern animals were shipped north and pastured with their northern counterparts, the northern animals would again begin to drop dead after about a month. When railway carloads of animals bound for slaughter in New York City began to die on the train, the industry began to panic.

Some western cattlemen suspected ticks, but to scientists in the waning years of the 1880s, the notion that an insect could cause infection was preposterous. In this new era of the germ theory, bacteria, not ticks, caused disease. But Smith, when he began investigating the problem, had the wisdom to listen to the farmers, not the scientists. He found that if he removed all the ticks from the southern cattle and then mixed those cattle with the northern herds, there was no disease. He also found that cattle that ate the ticks did not become sick, indicating that a tick bite was required. Furthermore, he discovered that it was the offspring of the ticks that were infectious; that was why there was a month's delay in the onset of illness. Last, he found tiny microorganisms in the red blood cells of the infected cattle.

Smith's experiments and subsequent publication of his discoveries in 1893 led to the practice of dipping cattle to "de-tick" them. This was an important practical result. More important, however, was the fact that this was the first time ever that an insect was shown to be the cause of a disease and transmission was by inoculation of an infectious agent by tick bite. This became a model for other important discoveries regarding the cause and control of African sleeping sickness, malaria, and yellow fever.

The Yale group began looking at many insects, but particularly ticks, to determine whether they were the vector for Lyme disease. Being careful and compulsive investigators, they went about this investigation the same way they had gone about the rest of the investigation. They assembled a group from Yale that included scientists from the Department of Epidemiology and Public Health, as well as other entomologists who were working in the area. They personally contacted all thirty-three physicians and the four visiting nurse associations practicing in the area as well as relevant specialists (such as dermatologists and rheumatologists) to identify as many patients with ECM or Lyme arthritis as possible.

In the summer and fall of 1977, they identified forty-three residents from twelve contiguous communities in Connecticut. Three of these towns—Old Lyme, Lyme, and East Haddam—were on the eastern bank of the Connecticut River. The other towns of Old Saybrook, Essex, Deep River, Chester, Haddam, Westbrook, Clinton, Killingworth, and Madison were located on the western bank. Now the goal of the investigators was to compare the incidence of disease on the east bank with that on the west bank. What Steere and Malawista found is that the disease was an astonishing thirty times more common on the east bank!

Another component of the study focused on ticks. Of the forty-three patients identified with Lyme disease, nine remembered being bitten by a tick at the site of the skin rash, usually within a week or two of the rash starting. Ticks were collected from the twelve communities on both sides of the Connecticut River. Small mammals were trapped, brought to the laboratory, anesthetized, bled, and examined for ticks. Most were returned to the wild. Deer that were shot in the normal course of the deer-hunting season were also examined when the hunters brought them into check stations. Some patients also brought in ticks.

The investigators found that *I. scapularis* nymphs were thirteen times more abundant on white-footed mice on the east bank compared with the west. They also found that the adult form of the tick was sixteen times more common on the east bank. Thus, both the incidence of the disease and the density of the tick were markedly increased on the same side of the river—the east bank—where the towns of Lyme and Old Lyme were situated. This clinched the notion that the tick was the vector; however, the attempt to recover and identify the causative agent of the disease still remained unsuccessful.

To understand vector-borne diseases, one must understand the trinity of *agent, vector,* and *reservoir.* These three components play out a delicate balance in nature independent of humans, who occasionally serve as an incidental host in this biological trinity. Typhus fever is a good example of this complex interrelationship and is best explained in Hans Zinsser's book *Rats, Lice and History.*

Although uncommon nowadays, typhus has played an enormous role in human history, often turning the tides of battles more than any general. Zinsser has estimated that thirty million people were infected with typhus and three million of those died between 1917 and 1923, the waning years and aftermath of the Great War. The agent is *R. prowazekii,* a rickettsia—those tiny bacterialike organisms that must live inside of cells. The vector (the organism that spreads the agent), is the body louse, which thrives in the overcrowded and unsanitary conditions associated with human disaster, hence its great role during war. The reservoir is the rat (and in some parts of the United States, the flying squirrel), whose role is to maintain the agent in nature, so that the vector can have an adequate supply.

Humans can play the role of reservoir, or host, too, if by accident the vector happens to interact with a human instead of a rat. In the case of typhus, it is not the bite from a louse that causes disease but scratching the louse on the skin. In this way, the blood of the louse, which contains the rickettsia, can gain access to the human and cause disease.

As of the late 1970s, the knowledge about this biological trinity of Lyme disease was growing: The agent was thought to be an infectious organism—either a virus or a penicillin-sensitive microbe—but its specific identity remained unknown. The vector was an *Ixodes* tick. The reservoir or natural host seemed to be the white-footed mouse and the white-tailed deer.

11 • An Intersection of Investigations

Tick-borne diseases, of course, were not new, and Dr. Steere and his colleagues at Yale weren't the only ones studying ticks and tick-borne diseases in the East; three other groups were actively pursuing investigations of tick-borne diseases. John Anderson and Louis Magnarelli (Figure 12), two entomologists from the Connecticut Agricultural Experiment Station (CAES) in New Haven, were primarily investigating cases of Rocky Mountain spotted fever (RMSF). Jorge Benach (Figure 13) was working as a pathologist with the New York Department of Health and was on staff at the State University of New York at Stony Brook. He was working on RMSF with Willy Burgdorfer (Figure 14) at the Rocky Mountain Laboratories (National Institutes of Health [NIH]) in Montana. Benach was also investigating babesiosis, a newer tick-borne infection that was increasing in incidence in the same area. There was some fear, later to be shown true, that babesiosis, a protozoan infection, could be transmitted by blood transfusion. For this investigation, he teamed up with Edgar Grunwaldt, the family practitioner on Shelter Island who first reported human babesiosis in New

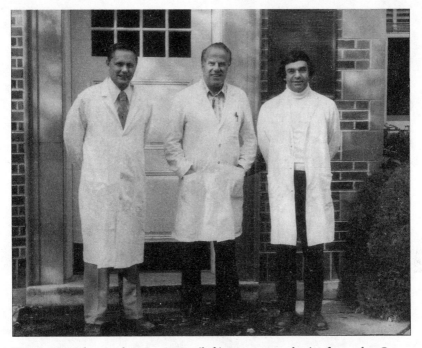

Figure 12. John Anderson, M.D. (left), an entomologist from the Connecticut Agricultural Experiment Station in New Haven, was investigating an increase in the East of Rocky Mountain spotted fever, another
tick-transmitted disease, with Dr. Louis Magnarelli (right) in the 1970s.
They sought out the expertise of Dr. Willy Burgdorfer (center) and eventually turned their attention to the tick that transmits Lyme disease.
(Photo from the late 1970s, courtesy of John Anderson, M.D., and Louis
Magnarelli, M.D.)

York State in 1977. Some of his patients seemed to have Lyme disease
and babesiosis at the same time.

The third group was headed by Dr. Andrew Spielman, of the
Harvard School of Public Health, who was already working in this
field at the time, investigating babesiosis on Nantucket Island. Gradually, these men and their stories began to intersect, and their work
on other tick-borne diseases would in time converge in the investigation of Lyme disease.

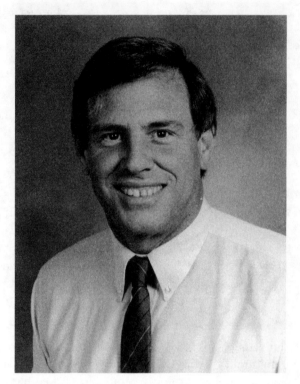

Figure 13. Jorge Benach, M.D., was working as a pathologist with the New York Department of Health and was on staff at the State University of New York at Stony Brook when his investigations of babesiosis and Rocky Mountain spotted fever placed him squarely in the investigation of Lyme disease. (Courtesy of Jorge Benach, M.D.)

According to Anderson, "1970 was an important year in the field of tick-borne diseases in the United States because two independent events were reported that year." That was the year that Milwaukee dermatologist Rudolph Scrimenti published his case report of the Wisconsin grouse hunter with a large red rash on his body at the site of a tick bite. The report, despite its brevity—barely more than one page—showed enormous presence of mind. For one thing, Scrimenti correctly recognized ECM even though it had never been reported

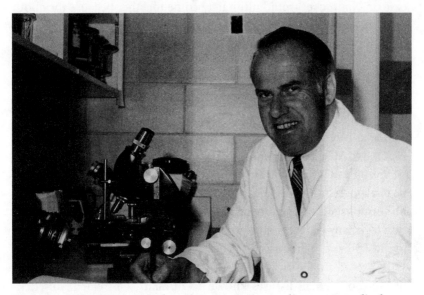

Figure 14. The bacterium found to cause Lyme disease, *Borrelia burg-dorferi,* was named after Dr. Willy Burgdorfer, who discovered the long-sought organism in 1981. (Photo from the 1980s, courtesy of Willy Burgdorfer, M.D.)

in a native North American. And like the Europeans, he successfully used penicillin to treat it. He even speculated on the etiology of this unknown malady—a spirochete—although he was unable to find any spirochetes when he examined biopsy specimens under the microscope.

Also in 1970 a group of physicians reported in the *New England Journal of Medicine* a case of human babesiosis in a patient with an intact spleen. Babesiosis is a parasitic disease quite similar to malaria. Before 1970, it was exceedingly rare in humans. Even more unusual, it had never been reported in patients with intact spleens because such people tended to be able to clear the babesia parasites from their systems.

Anderson says that these two milestones were important "because as it turned out, the tick disease in Wisconsin and the tick disease on Nantucket would ultimately come together because they both have the same vector. Different organisms, but the same vector, and they share the same reservoir—the white-footed mouse."

As we have seen, diseases can be passed, or vectored, to people in several ways; transmission by tick bite is one of them. As with many of the facts about Lyme disease in the United States, this one, too, was foreshadowed by observations in Europe. As early as the report by Afzelius in 1910, the European sheep tick, *I. ricinus,* had been implicated in the transmission of ECM. Numerous other European reports linking ECM, ACA, and lymphocytoma to tick bites had been published over many decades. The tick is the point of intersection for many different stories, and at this point, we turn to considering RMSF and babesiosis.

Spread by the rickettsial agent *R. rickettsia,* RMSF remains one of the most lethal diseases known to humans. Untreated, this tick-borne infection carries a mortality rate that approaches 40 percent. Its name derives from the fact that the disease first came to prominence in the Bitter Root Valley of Montana, where much of the original research on it was done. Even before European settlers began to flock to the area, drawn by the rich timber, Native Americans were aware of this disease. One tribe believed that evil spirits possessed these valleys, but only in the spring, although we do not know for sure that the fever was at the root of this legend. In the Shoshone tribe, most of the RMSF deaths occurred in the women because they went into the valleys each spring to chop and gather firewood.

As the area became increasingly populated with Europeans during the late 1800s, it was recognized that in the spring and summer, people regularly fell ill with a febrile illness marked by a prominent rash—red spots that started on the hands and feet and then spread to cover the entire body. Many died of what the settlers called "tick fever." By 1899, RMSF had been well-described by local physicians.

In 1906, Howard Taylor Ricketts, a pathologist from the University of Chicago, went to the Bitter Root Valley and initiated a series of experiments that were to be carried out over the next few years.

He first took the blood of patients with spotted fever and injected various fractions of the blood into laboratory animals. His findings, which were published in *JAMA,* showed that the plasma fraction (rather than the red or white blood cells, as had been the case with Theobald Smith's Texas cattle fever) could transmit the disease. If the plasma were filtered using a filter so fine that only a toxin or a virus would pass though it, then the filtered plasma could not transmit the disease. This suggested that the causative agent was large enough to be seen under the microscope, although to date, nobody had been able to accomplish this.

Further experiments using ticks that had fed on infected animals showed that the disease could also be transmitted by tick bite. In fact, this finding, by Ricketts and Walter King, was the first time that any human disease in the United States was shown to be transmitted in this fashion. Over the next few years, Ricketts worked out other details about the infectivity of ticks and showed that ticks in nature were infected and could transmit spotted fever to laboratory animals. The particular tick vector in the western states was *Dermacentor andersoni,* or the wood tick. The *Dermacentor* ticks are larger than the tiny *Ixodes* ticks and are the kind that many people are used to pulling off their pets.

Just like the people in the area around Lyme, Connecticut, the lumbermen in southwestern Montana were concerned that the increasing incidence of RMSF would negatively affect the price of real estate. The property value in the Bitter Root Valley was in jeopardy, especially on the west side of the valley, where the disease was more common. Furthermore, a huge enterprise organized by a group of Chicago financiers to irrigate the area in order to increase the McIntosh apple crop was also at risk. As Victoria Harden explains in her book *Rocky Mountain Spotted Fever: History of a Twentieth Century Disease:* "Spotted fever represented a distinct menace to this enterprise, which was expected to swell the population of the Bitter Root nearly tenfold as new orchards came under cultivation. Since scientific research had produced no cure and much confusion, local Bitter Root boosters adopted the tactic of officially ignoring the disease's existence. Beginning in 1904, newspapers rarely mentioned spotted fever in obituaries, usually describing it as fever or a brief illness."

In December 1909, Ricketts traveled to Mexico to study a form of typhus fever, whose vector had recently been shown to be the body louse. While his students continued his work on spotted fever, Ricketts became infected by the typhus germ and died from that disease on May 3, 1910. The group of organisms ultimately shown to cause both RMSF and typhus were of a novel type and were ultimately named in honor of Ricketts—the genus *Rickettsia*. Rickettsiae are distinguished from other bacteria in that they are obligate intracellular parasites (that is, they must live inside cells to survive) and are distinguished from viruses (which are also obligate intracellular organisms) by their much larger size and genetic makeup.

As the name Rocky Mountain spotted fever implies, this disease was thought to occur only in the western states. But in 1931 the first case was reported in the East, where the tick vector was *D. variabilis*, the common dog tick. The disease, however, had been around on the East Coast longer than that.

In 1991, a pathologist from the Johns Hopkins School of Medicine, J. Stephen Dumler, reported on a case of RMSF that he retrospectively diagnosed by restaining tissue specimen slides made ninety years earlier. Dumler found incontrovertible proof of RMSF in a patient seen on May 5, 1901. The treating physician was no less than the renowned Sir William Osler, who helped create the Johns Hopkins medical school and wrote *Principles and Practice of Medicine*, a definitive contemporary textbook of medicine. Osler diagnosed typhus fever. The next day, at the patient's autopsy, William Welch, an equally renowned pathologist in his day, described a rash that would have been consistent with typhus or RMSF. When Dumler restained the ninety-year-old paraffin-fixed tissue that Welch had prepared, this time for specific immunological stains specific for *R. rickettsia*, he showed that the rash was from RMSF.

This illustrates an important point. In medicine, one cannot diagnose what one does not know exists. Even as skilled a physician as William Osler could make such a mistake. Doctors on the eastern tip of Long Island had spoken of "Montauk knee" and "Montauk spider bite" for decades before the outbreak in Lyme, Connecticut. In retrospect, these patients almost certainly had Lyme disease. The case also demonstrates how the geographic range of a disease can change—another factor that was beginning to be seen with Lyme disease.

Rocky Mountain spotted fever propelled John Anderson of the CAES into the tick business. Over the ensuing decades since Ricketts's work, the incidence of RMSF had decreased in the mountain states and become more common in the south central and southeastern states. Today, Oklahoma and the Carolinas are the most common places to find the disease. But it was also present in the Northeast. In 1969, a report in the *New England Journal of Medicine* documented thirteen cases of RMSF diagnosed in Massachusetts residents, mostly from Cape Cod but also from the offshore islands of Martha's Vineyard and Nantucket. Two patients died.

Several years later, epidemiologists at the CDC were documenting an increase in the incidence of RMSF that was occurring over several years and seemed to be a trend. In the mid-1970s Anderson and Magnarelli began working in Old Lyme, Connecticut, because of a case or two of RMSF there. Working with rickettsiae was not easy and was potentially dangerous. Laboratory technicians working with *R. rickettsia* have occasionally become infected. The scientists from the CAES contacted colleagues at Yale, but nobody at the New Haven facility was working with rickettsiae; therefore, Anderson and Magnarelli had to learn the techniques themselves. They invited Dr. Burgdorfer to Connecticut so that he could show them some of these techniques. They also traveled to Hamilton, Montana, to learn other techniques at the Rocky Mountain Laboratories, which had been established in the 1930s as a local headquarters for investigating rickettsial diseases.

Anderson recalls traveling with all sorts of equipment: "I remember carrying it through O'Hare airport [in Chicago]. We had a lot of stuff." But it was worth it. "The result of all this ultimately ended up in the first isolation of *R. rickettsia* from a human case here in Connecticut, and that work was published."

During those same years, the mid-1970s, other researchers in New York were also studying RMSF. Jorge Benach was studying not only babesiosis, but also RMSF because there had been an increase in the mortality of the disease on Long Island. He teamed up with Burgdorfer, too, because of Burgdorfer's long history in dealing with tick-borne diseases, including rickettsial diseases. In 1975, Benach also traveled to Hamilton to learn the intricacies of working with rickett-siae. It wasn't entirely an accident that both groups—Anderson and Magnarelli from Connecticut and Benach from New York—ended up contacting Burgdorfer.

There simply weren't many men with Burgdorfer's experience left in the United States, and to some extent, in the world. Research required dollars, and with modern medical research shifting into the fields of cell biology and molecular genetics, money for research on ticks, spirochetes, and rickettsiae was drying up. Not only was government money evaporating, but commercial companies were getting out of the business of manufacturing vaccines for which there was little demand. Worst yet, because of these facts, very few young scientists were going into the field. Rickettsial diseases were thought to be a thing of the past.

But a funny thing happened to RMSF on its way to obscurity. Physicians still active with surveillance began to notice an increase in the number of cases, beginning in 1970. On Long Island, in Suffolk and Nassau counties, Benach was seeing this phenomenon, and so he and Burgdorfer began to study the problem. In 1977, they published a paper called "Changing patterns in the incidence of Rocky Mountain spotted fever on Long Island (1971–1976)." Of the 124 cases they described, eight patients died. Benach and his colleagues thought that some of this increase in incidence was due to changes in population patterns, a phenomenon that had been predicted as early as 1959. Areas that had once been duck and pumpkin farms were being transformed into trendy towns where people built homes and vacationed.

Some researchers in the area thought that there was a small increase in the percentage of fatal cases. Benach regularly sent ticks to Burgdorfer in Hamilton for analysis to see whether he and other researchers at Rocky Mountain Laboratories could find a reason for this phenomenon, but they came up empty-handed.

Simultaneously, Benach, as well as Anderson and Magnarelli, began looking into babesiosis, a malaria-like disease caused by a single-celled protozoan. Benach was trying to learn more about the possibility of blood transfusion–associated babesiosis, and in doing so, he maintained a serum bank of all the cases of babesiosis from Grunwaldt's patients on Shelter Island. The CAES entomologists' interest in babesiosis came from two directions. The first was that human cases were beginning to be described in the Northeast; the second was that Anderson became involved in an unusual case of babesiosis in a dog at about that time. "It was . . . a dog that lived in Connecticut but summered out on Cape Cod," recalls Anderson. The dog fell ill in June 1978 with fever and anemia. "The veterinarian out there did his own blood work," Anderson says. "And he saw organisms in the blood of this dog and thought it was babesia." Anderson and Magnarelli ultimately identified a babesia species never before seen in the United States—*B. gibsoni,* a species found in Africa and Asia. They published this investigation, "Canine *Babesia* New to North America," in the prestigious journal *Science* in 1979. Anderson thinks the parasites entered the United States in ticks that were hitching rides on the backs of pythons, boa constrictors, and dogs imported from South Africa.

Scientific advancement frequently comes from areas unrelated to the ultimate advancement. These men were scientists in the classic sense of the word—they were curious about the world around them, and they often pursued experiments simply for the sake of satisfying this curiosity. Many times these experiments led to dead ends, sometimes they would pay off immediately, and occasionally they would pay off indirectly in ways the researchers could not have planned or imagined.

Through all their investigations, Anderson and Magnarelli gained experience working with ticks, the parasites that live within ticks, and the various reservoirs (mice and other small mammals) for these parasites. And so when Lyme disease became a recognized entity, it was only natural that they began looking for its causative agent. From experience, they learned that peanut butter and seeds made good bait for mice, whereas raccoons preferred sardines. They learned how to catch, anesthetize, obtain blood from, and then release these animals back into the wild. The two entomologists had faculty appointments at Yale and were allowed to work in Dr. Robert Shope's lab. They performed these experiments on the *Ixodes scapularis* tick to try to find a virus, bacteria, or any other new organism that might be the cause of Lyme disease. But they found nothing.

Of course, dogs aren't the only species to suffer from babesiosis. In 1970 a group of physicians reported in the *New England Journal of Medicine* the case mentioned above of human babesiosis in a patient with an intact spleen. On July 13, 1969, a fifty-nine-year-old previously healthy woman was admitted to a New Jersey hospital after two weeks of fever, headache, abdominal cramps, and anemia. She had traveled in May from her home in Santa Barbara, California, to Nantucket Island, where she and her pet dachshund summered. She regularly pulled ticks off the dog, and on one occasion, she pulled a tick off herself.

The case report is rich with detail about her surroundings: "Mice were plentiful in the patient's frame cottage on the island. Her dog often chased, killed, and returned mice or other small rodents to the house. Because ticks were more common in this region than in California, the patient examined the dachshund daily and removed a number of ticks with tweezers or her fingers. In mid-May, she found a tick deeply embedded in her own suprasternal notch [where the collarbones and the breastbone meet] and removed it with some difficulty."

When she fell ill, she heeded the advice of a fellow vacationer, a doctor from New Jersey, and traveled the next day to New Brunswick, New Jersey, where she was immediately hospitalized. Because a blood smear suggested malaria, she was started on antimalarial drugs. But as she had never left the country, the smears were sent to the CDC, which confirmed that this was not malaria, but babesiosis.

A spleen scan confirmed that she had an intact, functioning spleen. She improved with chloroquine, a drug used for both protozoan infections.

After this first case of babesiosis described on Nantucket Island, Dr. Andrew Spielman began to study the ecology of that island. Initially, he wasn't terribly interested in the disease. "I was working mainly on mosquitoes," he remembers, "and I figured, well it's an oddity out there; it's a one-time thing that won't happen again." But then a neighbor of the Nantucket woman became infected.

The early 1970s was a time when governmental funding for science was being reduced, so Spielman was a bit hamstrung for funds. He remembers traveling to the island by ferry and then riding a bicycle from the boat pier to the town with "an enormous mountain of traps all over our bikes, each of us, the technician, his girlfriend, and myself loaded with the most inappropriate traps—raccoon traps. We had no idea, and we ended up on a cobblestone road . . . with traps falling off the bikes. It was just a mess." But Spielman persisted and was able to organize some local funding from the doctors on the island and the woman who had had the first case of babesiosis. "And so with the magnificent sum of $800, we started working on trying to figure out what was happening."

Then in 1977, Edgar Grunwaldt reported the first case of human babesiosis in a patient from Shelter Island. Therefore, as of the late 1970s, there were two new outbreaks of tick-borne infections—babesiosis and Lyme disease—in the Northeast, as well as concern about an increase in the incidence of a third—RMSF. The causal agent and treatment were known for babesiosis and RMSF. For Lyme disease, however, nobody had yet identified the agent, and there was considerable disagreement about the best treatment. These two stories—the cause and how it should be treated—are also intertwined. To best understand the search for the agent of Lyme disease, once again we must travel many decades back in time and recross the Atlantic.

12 • From the Alps to the Rockies

Willy Burgdorfer is a vigorous man with a prominent forehead, a large square jaw, thick white hair, and the handshake of a man many decades his junior. When he speaks, one can still hear a trace of a Germanic accent, despite the fact that he moved from Switzerland to the United States some fifty years ago.

In 1946, Dr. Rudolph Geigy, a professor of zoology at the University of Basel, Switzerland, accepted Burgdorfer as a graduate student at the Swiss Tropical Institute. Here, Burgdorfer was to develop his interest in the role of blood-sucking arthropods in the pathogenesis of both human and animal disease. Like many scientists after the Second World War, Burgdorfer and Geigy were studying issues important to the military, which often defined the destination of research dollars. Outbreaks of Q fever, another rickettsial illness, were affecting Allied troops throughout Europe, including in Switzerland. Burgdorfer and Geigy unsuccessfully looked for the agent in various arthropods. Despite their lack of success, Burgdorfer asked his professor whether he could work on a related project for his graduate work.

According to an account Burgdorfer wrote in 1993, Geigy responded by picking up a glass dish filled with light brown soil and said, "No problem. This sand contains several dozens of *Ornithodoros moubata* I collected in the Belgian Congo in 1945. As you know, this tick is the vector of the relapsing fever spirochete, *Borrelia duttonii*. Your thesis objectives will be to (1) establish a productive colony for spirochete-free ticks, (2) infect ticks with *B. duttonii* and study its development in the various tissues . . . and (3) identify the modes of transmission by immature and adult ticks."

Burgdorfer spent the next three years dissecting thousands of ticks to prepare tissue smears and sections. He then examined these specimens under the microscope, using both conventional and dark-field microscopy, a technique that venereal disease specialists had used to identify the syphilis spirochete. Dissecting thousands of ticks and examining their tissues led Burgdorfer to develop a new way of determining whether a tick was infected—an examination called the hemolymph test.

Tiny though they are, ticks have rudimentary alimentary, reproductive, nervous, and cardiovascular systems. They have mouth parts and salivary glands, intestines, and an exit from their alimentary tract. They have reproductive organs and a central ganglion, that is, a primitive nervous system. They also have hemolymph, which functions something like our blood, transporting nutrients to various parts of the tick.

"The rather consistent presence of *B. duttonii* in the hemolymph of infected ticks," wrote Burgdorfer, "led to the development of the hemolymph test as a relatively simple, rapid, and dependable technique to determine the prevalence of spirochete-infected ticks collected from nature. With this technique a small drop of hemolymph, obtained by cutting off the most distal portion of one or more legs, was examined microscopically for spirochetes. It proved to be the answer to Professor Geigy's frequent request to determine the prevalence of infected ticks from various sites in Tanzania."

To prepare for his doctoral thesis, Burgdorfer had to thoroughly familiarize himself with the medical literature on tick-transmitted spirochetal illnesses. Most of this literature related to relapsing fever, a borrelial infection spread by either a tick or a louse. When transmitted by tick, the tick species always belonged to the Argasidae, or soft ticks. The single exception Burgdorfer noted was *B. theileri*, the borrelial agent that causes a spirochetal disease of cows.

At the time, Burgdorfer was vaguely aware of the notion of several European dermatologists that ECM was a tick-transmitted spirochetal disease caused by the bite of *I. ricinus*. A few years later, the Swiss researcher also became aware of Hellerstrom's presentation at the Forty-Third Annual Meeting of the Southern Medical Association in Cincinnati, Ohio, in 1949, where Hellerstrom had raised the question of whether ticks are carriers of spirochetes. But Burgdorfer also realized that "there was no evidence to support that spirochetes were involved in ECM [Lennhoff's work never having been substantiated], and no one had ever found them [spirochetes] in the sheep tick, *I. ricinus,* or in any other species of this genus."

After Burgdorfer graduated in 1951, a research grant from Switzerland and a U.S. Public Health Service Fellowship allowed him to continue his studies at the Rocky Mountain Laboratories in Hamilton, Montana, under the sponsorship of Dr. Gordon E. Davis, the world's best-known borreliologist. Here, Burgdorfer continued his work on ticks and spirochetes, working with tick colonies that Davis maintained of thirteen different species of *Ornithodoros* ticks, each of which was parasitized by thirteen different species of *Borrelia*. However, the research did not proceed as he had hoped. At the Fortieth Annual Meeting of the International Northwestern Conference on Diseases in Nature Communicable to Man, held in August 1985, Burgdorfer explained why: "Unfortunately, by that time [December 1953], administrative interest in and support for research on relapsing fevers and tick-borne spirochetoses had completely vanished. I never will forget the discussion I had with Dr. Victor Haas, the director of the National Microbiological Institute (as we were then called): 'Relapsing fever,' he said, 'is a disease of the past; it no longer represents a public health problem. We cannot justify financial support for conducting research on an illness that each year may affect a handful of people who can be treated effectively with antibiotics. Considering your plans to stay on at RML [Rocky Mountain Laboratories], I strongly urge you to change to a different field of research.' Thus, work on tick-borne spirochetes, for me at least, became a moon-lighting job."

Getting out of the spirochete business made good administrative sense, even if it was not in the best interest of pure science. Eventually, other world-class institutions followed the lead of the Rocky Mountain Laboratories and moved on to other, more relevant diseases.

But reports of the death of relapsing fever were, as Mark Twain put it concerning his own reported death, "greatly exaggerated." Every so often, Burgdorfer would receive a call like one in March 1968 from Dr. Robert Thompson, a CDC EIS officer investigating an outbreak of a febrile illness among Boy Scouts who had camped out on Browne's Mountain, just southwest of Spokane, Washington. Burgdorfer was skeptical of the leading diagnosis at the time—Colorado tick fever—because of the elevation where the Scouts were camping (thirty-one hundred feet) and the fact that snow was still on the ground at the time the Scouts fell ill. Colorado tick fever, caused by a virus transmitted by the *D. andersoni* tick, is rarely contracted in areas at elevations of less than four thousand feet. Furthermore, Burgdorfer knew that the disease usually occurred during the warmer months of the year.

He therefore suggested to Thompson that they look for spirochetes in the blood smears of some of the patients. The smears were positive for borreliae, confirming Burgdorfer's suspicion that the patients actually had relapsing fever. Then in 1973, sixty-two people fell ill after spending several nights in a cabin on the North Rim of the Grand Canyon. Again, after a thorough epidemiological and clinical investigation, relapsing fever was found to be the culprit.

The genus *Borrelia* is one classification within the family of spirochetes and are so named after Amedee Borrel, a microbiologist at the Pasteur Institute of Paris. One disease they cause is relapsing fever, and the association of this kind of spirochete in the blood with relapsing fever was one of the first associations of a specific disease with a specific microbe. A German physician, Dr. Otto Obermeier, made this observation in 1868 while studying the blood of patients with relapsing fever during an epidemic in Berlin. His mentor, the famous pathologist Rudolph Virchow, did not allow the younger physician to publish his finding because he was unable to infect laboratory animals. Obermeier had to wait five more years for the next epidemic of relapsing fever. This time, he tried, unsuccessfully, to infect himself with the blood from a patient. Obermeier later performed another experiment on himself, this time with cholera. Two weeks later, he died.

Ten years later, Gregor Münch first proposed the idea that relapsing fever might be spread by blood-sucking arthropods, a theory later confirmed by French microbiologists in 1910. These Europeans were mainly dealing with the louse-borne form of relapsing fever. For the most part, the European form of the fever differed in its vector compared with the variety that British physicians Joseph Dutton and John Todd were studying in the Congo at the turn of the last century. This disease, the same one that Burgdorfer and Geigy were studying, was tick-borne. While performing an autopsy, Dutton accidentally infected himself and died from relapsing fever. Death-by-disease-that-one-was-studying was an all-too-common occupational hazard among medical scientists in the preantibiotic era! Dutton is remembered by the name *Borrelia duttonii*.

Also playing a role in research on relapsing fever was the great German physician and microbiologist Robert Koch. He was the first to demonstrate that spirochetes were transmitted via eggs (transovarial transmission) to the progeny of infected female ticks. But Koch's contributions to relapsing fever were minor compared with his other scientific achievements. Almost single-handedly, Koch drove the science of medicine across an enormous divide of thought, ushering in the age of bacteriology.

Koch was born in 1843 in northern Germany and received his medical degree twenty-three years later from the University of Göttingen. After the Franco-Prussian War of 1870, he began working as a district physician in a rural section of East Prussia called Wollstein. There, he became mired in the rigorous demands of a rural practice, without much leisure time to be stimulated by the numerous important scientific discoveries that regularly punctuated those decades.

Koch suffered from wanderlust, a habit his wife greatly wished to discourage, so for his twenty-eighth birthday, she bought him a microscope. The discoveries that he was to make with this microscope would ultimately take him on more journeys, both in the microscopic world and across the globe, than he or his wife could ever have imagined.

He began examining specimens from animals that had died from anthrax, a disease primarily of animals that was creating an enormous problem for farmers in northern Germany. He started seeing rod-shaped objects in the spleens of animals that had died of anthrax, but never in the spleens of animals that had died from other causes. He then tried to grow this rod-shaped object, which he presumed to be a bacterium, in his laboratory on an artificial medium. For that medium, he used the fluid from the anterior chamber of ox eyeballs, which also turned out to be an excellent growth medium for the anthrax bacillus.

Next, he inoculated these artificially grown bacilli into healthy mice and found that they died from anthrax. Finally, he examined the spleens of these animals that had died of the artificially grown anthrax bacilli and found the organism there, too. Koch achieved all of this in a tiny self-built laboratory in his home, using equipment that he privately financed on his meager salary. He presented his findings to leading German scientists in Breslau in 1876, and his career was launched.

He followed the anthrax project with an even more ambitious one: to elucidate the cause of tuberculosis, which killed one in every seven Europeans at the time. But first, Koch had to develop an artificial medium upon which to grow the bacteria—something more portable and easier to use than the fluid from the anterior chamber of an eye from a freshly killed ox. He experimented and experimented. He found that although beef broth mixed with a gelatin worked quite well for some bacteria, the tuberculosis bacillus would not grow at all on it. Koch tried various concentrations of the broth; he incubated them at different temperatures. He spent countless hours searching for the right combination. Finally, he hit upon a mixture of blood serum from freshly slaughtered cattle that worked for the tuberculosis germ.

And even with this concoction, he discovered that he needed to wait more than two weeks for the bacillus to grow, far longer than the time needed for any other bacteria he had ever worked with. This provided a valuable lesson in patience, as he had almost discarded these samples, thinking the experiment was a failure. These lessons would prove important, not just to Koch, but also to the generations of physicians who followed him.

Thus, one of Koch's contributions was to devise artificial media on which to grow germs outside of a diseased animal or patient. For some organisms, such as the anthrax bacillus, this was easy; for others, such as the tubercle bacillus, it was comparatively difficult. And for other organisms, such as the spirochete that caused syphilis, it has been, to the current day, impossible.

Koch also is known for the so-called Koch's postulates (sometimes referred to as the Koch-Henle postulates). As a meticulous and cautious researcher, Koch felt that simply culturing an organism from a sick individual was not sufficient to conclude that that organism caused that disease. Instead, he felt that four conditions must be met to make such a bold conclusion:

1. The specific organism should be shown to be present in all cases of animals suffering from a specific disease but should not be found in healthy animals.
2. The specific microorganism should be isolated from the diseased animal and grown in pure culture on artificial laboratory medium.
3. This freshly isolated microorganism, when inoculated into a healthy laboratory animal, should cause the same disease seen in the original animal.
4. The microorganism should be reisolated in pure culture from the experimentally infected animal.

Koch also discovered the comma-shaped cholera bacillus using these same techniques. It was Koch's statement that the comma bacillus was both necessary and sufficient to cause cholera that led Pettenkofer to imbibe the famous cholera-laden drink to try to disprove Koch. Koch's results with cholera also led to the vindication of John Snow's proclamation about the nature of the transmission of cholera some thirty years before. Unfortunately, Snow died twenty-five years before Koch's discovery.

Nature does not always reveal its secrets on a timetable that is advantageous to medical researchers, and such was the case with Snow regarding the laboratory cultivation of the cholera bacillus. In an era when Koch and others were cultivating the germs of anthrax, tuberculosis, cholera, gonorrhea, pneumonia, and dozens of other diseases, nobody had been able to do the same with the germ of relapsing fever. The best that investigators at the turn of the century could do was to keep borreliae alive by passing the bacteria into rodents and then harvesting the borreliae from the rodents' brains when they died— hardly a convenient method. In 1906, two researchers described a method for keeping borreliae alive that was only slightly less cumbersome—placing the bacteria in bags made from permeable membranes that contained serum which in turn were placed in the abdominal cavities of rabbits. This method allowed the researchers to confirm that borreliae could live outside animal cells. Others tried growing the spirochetes in chick eggs, but the science of cultivating borreliae in the laboratory on artificial medium did not advance much until 1971.

In that year, Richard Kelly, a pathologist working in Tennessee, reported on his method of growing borreliae outside live animals and on an artificial medium. Kelly succeeded where others failed because he added to his medium an ingredient that he suspected was important to the complex life cycle of borreliae, which spent a good portion of their existence inside ticks. He included in his recipe a specific amino sugar called N-acetylglucosamine. He made this addition because a polymer of this sugar forms chitin, which is an important part of the tick microenvironment. He reasoned that the borreliae might favor it. And he was right.

Three years later, Herbert Stoenner at the Rocky Mountain Laboratories performed more experiments culturing borreliae with this medium, which he later fortified with a variety of other ingredients such as yeast, amino acids, vitamins, and other growth factors. Therefore, just a few years before everyone started looking for the causative agent of Lyme disease, a method for culturing borreliae was finally available.

13 • To Treat or Not to Treat?

Normally, doctors know how to best treat a disease only after they know what causes it. For Lyme disease, however, that sequence was reversed. As of the late 1970s, two clear schools of thought competed with respect to the therapy of Lyme disease. As we have already seen, the Navy doctors from Groton, Mast and Burrows, strongly believed in antibiotics, and European dermatologists routinely treated with antibiotics the three types of rashes thought to be related—ECM, ACA, and lymphocytoma. The Yale group, on the other hand, considered Lyme disease to be due to a virus, which would not require treatment with antibiotics. Because the Yale group was doing most of the clinical research at this point, other clinicians were influenced by their opinion. For example, Edgar Grunwaldt, who had initially begun treating his patients with antibiotics when he first arrived at Shelter Island, stopped doing so in 1978 after Steere assured him that the disease was self-limiting.

Nevertheless, Steere, Malawista, and the others from Yale recognized the opposite point of view as well as the weight of evidence from the other side of the Atlantic. They wanted to get it right, so they set up a simple trial. They decided to treat everybody in 1977 with antibiotics and then, in 1978, to withhold antibiotics. They felt that after they analyzed the data from the two summers, the imperative to treat or not with antibiotics would be clear.

When this situation is seen through the all-powerful "retrospectoscope," it might look as if the need for antibiotics was obvious. But oftentimes, that which appears obvious with the passage of time is not nearly so clear in the beginning. Many diagnostic tests and therapies have been incorporated into medical practice over the years that, at the time they were introduced, had some face validity, or "obvious" truth. That is, they made sense pathophysiologically, or they agreed with the conventional wisdom. Sometimes, however, they fail to hold up to the scrutiny of a well-designed scientific trial. Some of the data available for Lyme disease, especially the human transmission experiments of Erich Binder for ECM and Hans Gotz for ACA, seemed to cinch the existence of a transmissible agent. But such experiments did not prove that the transmissible agent was sensitive to antibiotics.

A purist would argue that these earlier experiments were not performed on enough subjects. That same purist would also argue that a control group should have been included; that is, the German researchers should have taken a skin biopsy from a patient with ECM or ACA and then inoculate a larger group of volunteers. If most of the volunteers developed the rash, it would likely to be due to a transmissible agent; however, that would be consistent with a viral, or other nonantibiotic-sensitive, organism as well.

To deal with this problem, the purist's experiment would then treat half of the group of inoculated volunteers with antibiotics and withhold antibiotics from the other half. To be even more scientifically rigorous, the purist experiment would treat half with a placebo in a manner such that neither the doctor nor the patient knows who is receiving an antibiotic and who is receiving a placebo. This is called a double-blind, placebo-controlled study; both the patient and the doctor are "blind" to which treatment is being given.

One could argue that such an experiment is unethical; however, the ethics depend on how well-established a concept is before an experiment is done. Had the notion that antibiotic treatment was effective been 100 percent established in 1978, then such an experiment would have exposed its subjects to unnecessary danger. But if the concept really were not yet established, then the experiment would be justified in order to establish the fact. Nowadays, every hospital has an institutional review board that referees medical investigations and helps protect patients from unnecessary risk.

Some people think that everything doctors do is based on careful scientific experimentation and analysis and that their actions are always dictated by carefully constructed science. Unfortunately, this is simply not the case. Many diagnostic tests and treatments have been accepted as medical "gospel" despite the absence of any real scientific foundation. Then, once something has been established as a standard of care, it seems risky, or at least imprudent, to deviate from it. Sometimes, the condition to be studied is so rare that well-done, controlled experiments are difficult to organize. Other times, the condition may be sufficiently acute or rapidly progressive that there is no time to properly enroll patients or obtain proper informed consent. Still other times, finances define how medical research proceeds. Large pharmaceutical companies fund much of scientific research, and their goal is to earn profits for the company. If a drug or treatment has been available for a while and has no commercial support, research for that drug will not be funded.

Perhaps the most important reason that physicians' practices are not always formed on the underpinning of great science is the most insidious of all—human nature. Doctors get used to doing something one way; it becomes "generally accepted," a "standard of care," or the "prevailing wisdom" even if it has never been properly tested—and sometimes never will be.

This weakness of human nature is as prevalent among patients as doctors. As Osler put it, "the desire to take medicine is perhaps the greatest feature that distinguishes man from animals." Take the example of many self-limited upper respiratory infections—the common cold, or even acute bronchitis. Abundant data indicate that treating these conditions with antibiotics is unnecessary. And yet patients continue to demand them, so doctors continue to prescribe them. This fact is creating many problems. Aside from the financial costs, allergic reactions, and other medication side effects, probably the biggest concern is how we are now seeing an increase in "antibiotic-resistant" bacteria. Because most bacteria reproduce in hours, genetic mutations occur that defend against even the newest, most powerful antibiotics. Evolutionary pressure is highly efficient. One can blame the pharmaceutical companies for "pushing" newer, more expensive, broader spectrum antibiotics on the public, but the underlying responsibility rests with physicians and patients—in short, with our societal imperative for taking medication when we get sick.

Peptic ulcer disease is another recent example of how "prevailing wisdom" affected the course of research and therapy. Until the 1980s this common problem was universally thought to be due to factors such as stress, bad genes, spicy foods, and alcohol and tobacco use, which increased the acidity in the stomach, leading to ulceration of the stomach lining. Eliminate the stress, fix the diet, and treat the acid and ulcers should improve. And initially, they did. But six months after stopping the antacids, half of the patients relapsed, and by two years out, almost all of them did—not surprisingly, when the etiologic factors (stress, bad genes, and bad habits) were still present. Many of these patients ultimately underwent surgery to remove the ulcerous portion of the stomach or to cut the nerves that created the acidity in the first place. Ulcer surgery was common in the 1950s, 1960s, and 1970s.

Then an Australian internal medicine resident named Barry Marshall questioned this theory. Working with one of the hospital's pathologists, Dr. J. Robin Warren, he found a corkscrew bacterium in the area of the ulcer in eighty-seven of one hundred surgical or endoscopic specimens. Reviewing the literature, he found that articles had mentioned this finding as far back as 1893! He also found a 1940 study suggesting that the substance bismuth could cure ulcers.

Marshall thought that if he could culture the organism and show that bismuth inhibited its growth, then he would be partly on the way to showing that this bacterium—originally named *Campylobacter pylori* and later changed to *Helicobacter pylori*—caused ulcers. He spent months trying to grow the bacterium. Like Koch, he persisted in trying different culture media under different conditions, in experiment after experiment. Finally, over the long Easter weekend of 1982, he was successful, having left the plates of culture medium in the incubator for longer than the usual two days (he had almost forgotten Koch's lesson of patience). Then, he placed some bismuth on the culture plate and found that it inhibited the bacterial growth. Warren and Marshall's initial attempt to have their work published in *Lancet* was rejected; their hypothesis flew in the face of conventional wisdom.

Marshall then initiated a clinical trial of bismuth. Although patients treated with bismuth showed an initial good response, eventually most of them relapsed, just like those given antacids. Always the careful observer, Marshall noticed that one patient did not relapse; this patient had been given metronidazole, an antibiotic prescribed for a coincidental gum infection. He started this combination therapy and found that 70 percent of his patients improved and maintained that improvement.

At this point, some of the local television stations picked up the story. One man, who was scheduled for ulcer surgery the next morning, saw a newscast about the work Marshall was doing and telephoned him. The patient had gone so far as to sell his business on the advice of his doctors, who thought that the stress of his business had caused the ulcer. The night before the surgery, Marshall rushed to the hospital, passed an endoscope down the man's esophagus, found the bacteria, and treated him (without the surgery) with repeated courses of bismuth and antibiotics. He cured that man.

Marshall presented his data at medical meetings, but still nobody believed him. Everyone knew that bacteria didn't cause ulcers; after all, how could they withstand the acidity of the stomach? Finally, like so many before him, Marshall resorted to self-experimentation, drinking, like Pettenkofer, the very bacteria he had grown in the lab. Several days later, he fell ill with violent stomach pains and vomiting; he took the bismuth and antibiotic, and cured himself. It took many more years and many more rejections, both from colleagues and from some of the best medical journals in the world, before Marshall was vindicated.

There are numerous other examples—from the need for radical mastectomy in breast cancer to the use of special pulmonary artery diagnostic catheters with patients in intensive care units—that illustrate how the medical community frequently acts more on the basis of culture and tradition than on solid scientific evidence.

So how well-established was the notion that antibiotics could cure the various manifestations of Lyme disease? This question actually contains multiple questions. First, which antibiotics? Even in the mid-1970s, many antibiotics were available, and these were not equally effective against all types of microorganisms. Recall that bacteria have different outer cell membrane characteristics that stain differently with Gram's stain. Some antibiotics were more powerful against so-called Gram-positive organisms, whereas others seemed to have a greater effect against Gram-negative bugs. So choosing the wrong antibiotic could affect the outcome of experimentation. Second, what was the dosage, that is, how much antibiotic for how long? These two factors are important in many kinds of infections. If too low a dose is taken for the prescribed period of time, the infection may not be cured; but if the correct dose is taken for too brief a period of time, the infection may also not be cured.

Most important, in the late 1970s, the cause of Lyme disease was still unknown. This fact was a major impediment in the research on both diagnosis and treatment. If the cause were clearly known to be a virus, then antibiotics available in the late 1970s would have been ineffective. If on the other hand the causative agent were shown to be a bacterium, then the imperative to treat would be greater. Also, it was possible that the initial symptoms were caused by an unknown bacterium but the later manifestations, of arthritis for example, were caused by immunological mechanisms rather than active infection. Thus, antibiotics might cure one phase of the disease but be ineffective against another. At this point, the precise relationship between the rash and the arthritis, which had not been described even in the European literature, was still being explored.

All of these issues made it unclear to the Yale investigators how to best treat the disease. Remaining open-minded, however, they went ahead with their simple trial of treating with antibiotics one summer and not the next. There was no big meeting. Steere, despite the fact that he was still a junior member of the team, was given a great deal of independence in running the investigation. "Steve Malawista was my mentor," explains Steere. "And we talked about things frequently. And what's more, I think he has good judgment about whether something made sense or not. But the way he operates is he does allow people at least the potential for a lot of autonomy."

"It was after that summer's experience [1976] and talking with Drs. Mast and Burrows that I decided what we'd do next summer [1977]," Steere says. "So we would treat everyone with Penn G [penicillin] and follow them and see what happens." By "what happens," Steere meant that they would measure how fast the rash improved and how many of the patients went on to develop a secondary manifestation, such as nerve, heart, or joint problems. When they analyzed the data, they found that the ECM seemed to disappear more quickly in the antibiotic-treated patients, but they attributed some of this variation to what they termed the "variable natural course" of the disease. As of the end of the 1977 season, they still maintained that antibiotics were not indicated.

The next summer, the New Haven group once again decided to routinely withhold antibiotics. By the fall of 1978, having one more summer's worth of experience, the data seemed to indicate that antibiotics did help, enough so that in the summer of 1979, they again began to routinely prescribe antibiotics. After they analyzed the data from all four summers, the Yale doctors were clearly able to establish that antibiotics helped both to reduce the duration of ECM and to reduce the likelihood of subsequent manifestations.

Despite their initial bias, the Yale group concluded: "For patients with ECM, we recommend prompt treatment with oral penicillin for seven to 10 days. However, it is neither clear that penicillin is the antibiotic of choice nor that such dosage and duration of therapy is optimal. Our second choice is tetracycline for the same period, except for children below the age of eight because of the risk of tooth discoloration." They further acknowledged being unsure whether patients with later manifestations of Lyme disease should receive penicillin.

By now, the investigators were clearly developing the notion that the disease occurred in stages. The tick bite led to the skin rash ECM. Later, some patients went on to develop neurological, cardiac, and rheumatic manifestation. By this time also, cases from other parts of the United States had begun to crop up. Some were from the upper midwestern states, such as Wisconsin, where Scrimenti reported his first case in 1970. The other area was the West Coast—California and Oregon—where the tick vector was *I. pacificus,* a tick related to *I. ricinus* and *I. scapularis.*

Recall that Andrew Spielman and colleagues were pursuing investigations of babesiosis on Nantucket Island. The same tick species served as vector for both Lyme disease and babesiosis. During their investigations they began to notice differences in the ticks. Spielman thought that there were sufficient differences in the *Ixodes* ticks on Nantucket Island, and indeed all over the Northeast, that they were a different species from *I. scapularis,* which had been identified as the vector for Lyme disease. In 1979 he and colleagues published their work and renamed the vector of babesiosis (and Lyme disease) in the Northeast to *I. dammini,* in honor of the Harvard pathologist Gustav Dammin.

This change in nomenclature was not without its effect, for it meant that doctors could not "legitimately" make a diagnosis of Lyme disease in states where the vector was not found. If *I. dammini* (only prevalent in the Northeast) were a separate species from *I. scapularis* (whose northernmost range is the middle Atlantic states), then doctors would not be able to diagnose Lyme disease in the southern states. In 1979, Steere and Malawista published an article showing that cases of Lyme disease directly overlapped with areas where *I. dammini* was found in the Northeast and *I. pacificus* was found in the Northwest. And thus the reader will need to make this shift in nomenclature from *I. scapularis* to *I. dammini.*

14 • The Scramble for the Cause

At the same time as the Yale group was evaluating the utility of antibiotic therapy, they were also active in trying to find the culprit organism. "By 1979, we had come to think that this might really be a spirochetal illness," recalls Steere. "The main reason was that it was clear that ECM responded to antibiotics, to penicillin, and you had to put that together with an illness that occurred in stages. You know, here's the ECM, then later was the arthritis. And finally the histology [the structure under the microscope] always showed lymphocytes. I remember sitting down with Dick Root, who was the head of infectious diseases at the time, who said, 'You know, let's go through Bergey's manual, which lists every organism that is known, and let's apply these three criteria'—and so we did. We started off with staphylococci because that's what came first in the book, then we went to streptococci. Before too long, you come to the spirochetes—to the borrelia in the spirochetes section."

When Steere and Root got to *Borrelia,* they thought it fit better than anything else they had been looking at. Steere asked Root, " 'Well how do you culture a borrelia?' And he said, 'It's a real bitch.' "

The Yale people were working with the CDC, and Steere remembers that the head of the bacterial diseases division was not enthusiastic about the idea of culturing ticks: "He said, 'There's going to be a lot of stuff in them. You're going to have trouble with contamination. You're not going to be able to know what is what, and you'll have no idea of what percentage of them are infected.' On the other hand, you're postulating that the organism is in the ECM lesion. So we'll culture that, which we started doing in the summer of 1980. We decided to stay more on the patient side of things, figuring that this is our area and that the organism should be there."

So the Yale group developed a protocol in collaboration with the CDC to culture the skin lesions from patients with ECM. Steere's main contact at the CDC was another EIS officer named George Schmid, who was assigned to the bacterial zoonoses branch. Zoonoses are diseases in which animals play an important role in the transmission.

"When we decided to work together with Allen," Schmid recalls, "I didn't have a good feel for the disease. I really didn't know what it was like, other than reading or talking with Allen. So I decided to spend a week up in New Haven, and at that time, Allen had a Lyme disease clinic. So I went up there. Here I am at the height of the season probably about May of 1981, but not a single case of Lyme disease came in that week." However, a woman came into the clinic who had been seen there the week before. She described how, after she had taken the antibiotics, her fever went higher, accompanied with shaking, and her skin rash got redder. Schmid thought, "That sounds very much like a Jarisch-Herxheimer reaction. And so I said, what causes Jarisch-Herxheimer reactions? And the answer was, of course, spirochetes."

A Jarisch-Herxheimer reaction occurs during the initial hours after a spirochetal infection is treated. First described by Adolf Jarisch in 1895 and separately by Karl Herxheimer in 1902, the reaction followed the treatment of syphilis, which in those days was with mercury. Several hours after antibiotics are started, the patient begins to feel horrible; the fever spikes, and chills follow. The pulse quickens, and the rash, if there was one, intensifies. The blood pressure usually is alarmingly low, but then, without any real treatment, other than perhaps some fluids and time, the reaction passes as quickly as it came.

The Jarisch-Herxheimer reaction is thought to be due to the rapid destruction of the spirochetes, with a resultant release of various components of their cell membranes into the circulation. The body's immunological reaction to these foreign substances creates the reaction, which may follow treatment of syphilis, relapsing fever, and leptospirosis. So although Schmid left New Haven without having seen a case of Lyme disease, he had a vivid impression of this woman's symptoms—and yet another small piece to the complex puzzle suggesting that this was a spirochetal disease.

As the researchers investigated specimens from patients with Lyme disease, they looked "for all sorts of organisms—fungi, viruses, everything," Schmid says. "We inoculated material into eggs, into the brains of mice, and into tissue culture. To make a long story short, we looked carefully for spirochetes. We didn't want to miss a spirochete. And so we used leptospire medium and Kelly's medium looking for borrelia. Allen spent the summer of 1981 getting specimens— from skin, CSF [cerebrospinal fluid], whole blood—thinking that all of them would be potential sources for organisms, including spirochetes."

And they found a spirochete! "But it wasn't quite the spirochete I was hoping for," says Schmid. They found a leptospire, which is in the spirochete family. "Leptospirosis was different from Lyme disease; they were both spirochetal in nature but not really much alike. Nevertheless, it was the right type of organism. We then tried to figure out if it was the right one or not. So using acute and convalescent sera we developed an IFA test and tried to figure out if this was the bug or not."

An immunofluorescent antibody (IFA) test helps researchers see whether a patient is producing specific antibodies to a particular germ. Bacteria, viruses, fungi, and all living cells for that matter, are separated from the rest of the world by a cell wall or membrane. But the cell membrane does a lot more than just act as a barrier to the outside world; it has substance, shape, topography, and function. It is composed of a bilayer of complex fatty molecules called *phospholipids*. Mixed into this lipid layer, much like the chips in a chocolate chip cookie, are proteins, which act as channels through which some molecules are allowed entrance into the cell and others are not.

The shape and texture of this outer coat, the cell membrane, differs from organism to organism; that is, for instance, the outer membrane of a streptococcus is different from that of a spirochete. The more similar two organisms are, however, the more similar the textures of their cell membranes; so the textures of two different kinds of bacteria, such as the streptococcus and the spirochete, will share some commonality. Even within the different kinds of spirochetes, while there is increasingly more and more in common, there are also distinctions in their outer coats. So a borrelia will be different from a treponeme, which will be different from a leptospire.

Various regions on the outer coats serve as *antigens*. Simplistically speaking, antigens are a region of a cell, or even of a protein or other molecule, that has a particular shape and topography. *Antibodies* are also molecules, made by specific kinds of white blood cells called B-lymphocytes. Specific antibodies bind to the specific antigens, much like a key fits into a lock or a hand into a glove. But these molecules are just that—molecules, which is to say, they are far too small to see. Therefore, to be able to "see" the binding of antibodies and antigens and measure it, scientists attach markers onto the antibody molecule. In the late 1970s and early 1980s, the usual test was the IFA. Researchers would tag the antibody with another molecule, fluorescein, which would fluoresce and appear a brilliant copper-green color under the microscope.

The IFA test works something like this. The lab technician fixes the antigen (in Steere and Schmid's case, the leptospire that they found in the skin lesion) into a well on a glass slide. She then adds the antibody (from the Lyme disease patient's serum, which contains antibody and which has been tagged with fluorescein). If antibody from the serum matches the antigen on the slide, they will bind tightly together. The next step is to wash off with distilled water any loose antibody that didn't bind. Whatever is left on the slide is antibody (with the fluorescent marker) bound to antigen. The technician then looks under a microscope to see how much, if any, fluorescence is still visible on the slide.

As with many laboratory tests, however, results can vary, as there is always interpretation involved when the technician "reads" the slide. If there is no fluorescence, the test is unequivocally negative; but there could be a variable amount of fluorescence, which could be interpreted as "weakly" positive or "strongly" positive. Think about the key and glove analogies. Sometimes a key will fit into a lock but won't be precisely the correct key, as the door won't open. And sometimes a hand will fit into a glove but not exactly right, as the glove is a little too loose or too tight.

This is analogous to cross-reacting antibodies, that is, antibodies that partially "fit" more than one antigen. Some antigens on the outer coat of borreliae are sufficiently similar to those on leptospires (remember that they are closely related bacteria, both in the spirochete family) so that there is a partial fit. A little bit of the antibody binds to some antigen because it is almost the correct shape and size. The distilled water washes some of it away, but some of it remains on the slide, loosely bound to the antigen. You get what is called a weak reaction; there is some ambiguity in the result.

Another thing to know about the IFA test is the concept of a *titer*. What is being tested is how dilute a serum specimen can be and still show antibody to the antigen being investigated. The serum is mixed one-to-one with water (a titer of 1:2), and then this is mixed with an equal part of water (a titer of 1:4). As each dilution is progressively mixed with another equal part of water, the titers rise exponentially—1:8, 1:16, 1:32, 1:64, and so on. Higher numbers after the 1 indicate a stronger reaction, or a higher level of antibodies in the patient's serum.

Finally, one should understand the difference between acute and convalescent phase sera. Doctors look at serum taken from a patient at the very early stages of infection (the acute phase), before antibodies have had time to be produced; and then they look at serum taken several weeks later (the convalescent phase), after the antibodies have had time to form. If a specific antibody was absent in the acute phase serum and then present in the convalescent phase serum, this strongly suggests that the patient has been exposed to the organism within the preceding weeks.

The leptospire that Steere and colleagues isolated from an ECM skin lesion was one that was previously unidentified. "It never had been seen before on the face of the earth," Steere says. "It hasn't been ever since, either. And so we started testing serum against this leptospire. We knew that this was an undescribed organism and that it had come out of an ECM skin lesion, supposedly. And we were seeing reactivity with it. Though even with that, there was kind of a suggestion of cross-reactivity."

But the reactions in the lab that the scientists were seeing weren't definitive. The reaction when they placed patients' serum with the organism was not always predictable, or there was a weak reaction. After the serum was diluted a little, there was no reaction. Although it seemed that they were on the right track, at the same time, "there was the feeling that this wasn't quite right," says Steere.

Schmid has the same recollections: "We found that there was low-level reactivity in the convalescent sera in a number of the patients with Lyme disease; titers not that high. Although we were seeing serologic changes, they were not nearly of the magnitude we were hoping for. And all we had was the one, single isolate. We couldn't get it from other tissue samples. We also looked for it in tissue using silver stains, but we couldn't find it in the pathology [specimens]." The two investigators felt that although this didn't feel like the real thing, they still had indirect evidence that a spirochete was involved.

While the Yale and CDC team was trying to culture this new organism from the skin, other groups and individuals were also busy looking for the agent responsible for Lyme disease. The news from the United States regarding Lyme disease was exciting for the Europeans. Although ECM and ACA had existed in Europe for a century, the two diseases had never been the subject of this kind of focused, extensive research. Many of the secrets of ECM were yielding to this new blitz-

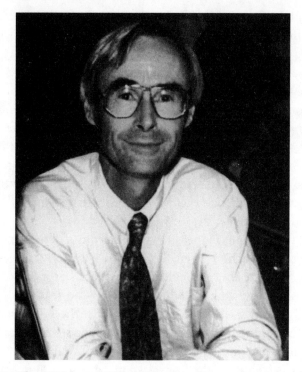

Figure 15. Klaus Weber, M.D., a German dermatologist, worked over several decades to discover the cause of erythema migrans (EM). (Courtesy of Klaus Weber, M.D.)

krieg of research. As trans-Atlantic collaboration increased, it became more and more apparent that although researchers on both sides of the ocean were dealing with the same disease, there were differences between the European and U.S. versions. For example, the erythema of the ECM rash did not seem to be as chronic in U.S. patients. Furthermore, the chronic skin rash ACA was almost never seen in the New World. And the frequency of some of the neurological and joint manifestations seemed to differ.

During the 1970s, even before the discovery in Lyme, one German researcher who was very active and interested in this field was Klaus Weber, a Munich dermatologist (Figure 15). As a practicing dermatologist in Bavaria, Weber was as up-to-date as anyone in the world on the subject of ECM, ACA, and lymphocytoma and was regularly treating patients with these conditions. As early as 1970, well before the Connecticut outbreak, he had undertaken some initial but unsuccessful attempts to find the organism.

Then in 1974, one year before Mrs. Murray and Mrs. Mensch called the Connecticut authorities, Weber published a case report of a woman with ECM and meningitis whom he successfully treated with antibiotics. Weber was well aware of Hellerstrom's work published in 1950, and based on his own additional case, he proposed that ECM-related meningitis was a bacterial infection, not a viral one. He considered *Borrelia* and *Rickettsia*. If not one of these, then he reasoned that this disease was caused by a hitherto unknown bacterial species.

As for *Rickettsia,* French investigators reported that in six of seven patients with ECM, they found high titers of antibodies against various rickettsial organisms, including the causes of typhus, murine typhus, and Mediterranean spotted fever (boutonneuse fever). Other French investigators found similar findings, but no other groups could ever reproduce these results. Nevertheless, the notion of a possible rickettsial etiology remained active. In fact, as late as 1979, there was a report of rickettsia-like organisms found by electron microscopy in macrophage cells (scavenger cells of the body) from two patients with ECM.

Weber also considered but rejected the possibility that borreliae were the culprit. There were two reasons for this. The first was that, Lennhoff's work on spirochetes in 1948 notwithstanding, many other dermatologists had searched for and failed to find spirochetes. Given the common roots of dermatology and the study of venereal diseases, the dermatologists were the most expert on syphilis and therefore were expert at looking for treponemes by dark-field microscopy. They had looked for spirochetes in ECM lesions and found none. Weber said, "I found it quite unlikely that so many dermatologists experienced in looking at dark-field preparations for *T. pallidum* were unable to detect spirochetes in ECM lesions; often, it is better to know nothing."

The second reason why Weber thought borrelia unlikely was another bit of conventional wisdom that turned out to be wrong. In a 1965 review on borrelia Weber read that "ticks propagating human relapsing fever belong to the Argasidae [soft ticks], never to the Ixodidae [hard ticks]." *I. ricinus*, the vector in Europe, was a hard, Ixodid tick. But still, Weber maintained that the cause must be an antibiotic-sensitive, unknown bacterium.

Weber persisted in his search for that bacterium. In 1978, he approached a bacteriologist at the Pettenkofer Institute in Munich. "I sent her skin biopsy material from several of my patients but she failed to isolate any agent," Weber remembers. "Unfortunately, she did not use the Kelly medium, which had been known at that time for about four years." He also asked that some of the material be stained with a special silver stain, called Dieterle's stain, but the person in the lab used a different, unreliable stain.

Dr. Rudolph Ackermann (Figure 16) was another German researcher who had been searching for the cause of Lyme disease. A neurologist, he was at the forefront of the European efforts to define the syndrome known as Bannwarth's syndrome. In 1973, he and colleague Dr. Peter Horstrup reported on forty-seven patients that Ackermann had seen from 1956 to 1972 with the painful syndrome of meningoradiculitis (inflammation of the meninges and nerve roots)—the syndrome that Bannwarth had described in 1941 as well as Garin and Bujadoux in the 1920s before that.

During this time before computerized databases were generally available, a literature search was a real gumshoe operation. "On our difficult search through the libraries for publications about the disease called Bannwarth's syndrome and related manifestations," Ackermann recalls, "my coworker Peter Horstrup would exhume in a library in Paris in the *Journal de Medecine de Lyon* of Charles Garin and Bujadoux with the title 'Paralysie par les Tiques.' This brilliant and [revealing] case report was forgotten for forty years, presumably because it was published in a local medical journal and because the title for the disease generally is used for another tick-borne illness." This report therefore had lain for decades undiscovered. But because of this "rediscovered" connection, Horstrup and Ackermann referred

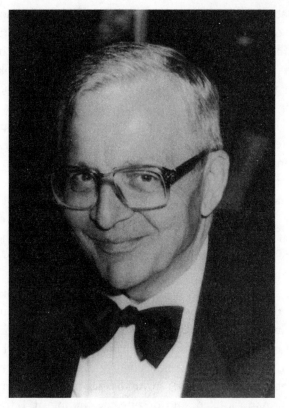

Figure 16. Rudolph Ackermann, M.D., a German neurologist, worked for decades to uncover the cause of Bannwarth's syndrome. (Courtesy of Rudolph Ackermann, M.D.)

to this disease of a lymphocytic meningoradiculitis as Garin-Buja-doux-Bannwarth's syndrome.

From the perspective of a neurologist, especially one practicing during the 1950s through the 1970s, a virus seemed to be the likeliest cause for this syndrome. Other prominent European neurologists, such as Georges Schaltenbrand, had presumed this to be the case. Ackermann searched for one diligently: "Schaltenbrand's first presumption that Bannwarth's syndrome could be caused by the FSME [a virus that causes encephalitis—an inflammation of the brain] was not probable because of the different clinical picture. Also, we were unable to demonstrate FSME antibodies in the serum of patients with Bannwarth's syndrome. Holstrom's observation of a case of EM and meningitis successfully treated with penicillin was overlooked or neglected by most of the neurologists. Because of the lymphocytic meningitis, the normal temperature [and blood tests], and the self-limited course of Bannwarth's syndrome and of EM, they believed it to be of a viral etiology.

"Ironically, in 1970, we had been able to isolate a new virus called Tettnang virus from ticks collected at three different sites where patients had been bitten by ticks and then developed Bannwarth's syndrome. This finding seemed to confirm our hypothesis of the viral etiology of Bannwarth's syndrome. But all efforts to find the etiologic relation of Tettnang virus with patients with Bannwarth's syndrome ended without success."

The seasonal pattern of the disease and the occasional association with tick bite all fit with an arthropod mechanism, but was also compatible with a virus, just as Steere had initially reasoned in the United States. In Europe, there was already a disease model for this— tick-borne encephalitis, an inflammatory disease of the central nervous system caused by a virus spread by tick bite. But no matter how hard Ackermann looked, and despite the finding of Tettnang virus in ticks, he could not find a virus in the patients with Bannwarth's syndrome.

In the United States, John Anderson and Lou Magnarelli had turned from their investigations into RMSF and were also looking for the agent that caused Lyme disease. They trapped animals in the areas where Lyme disease was common—Lyme and East Haddam— removed any ticks that they found, and then examined the ticks for microorganisms. Jorge Benach in New York also turned his focus from RMSF to Lyme disease, working with Dr. John Hanrahan, another EIS officer, assigned to the New York State Health Department in 1981. As in the original Lyme outbreak that Dr. Snydman had detailed, these investigators were finding that within counties where Lyme disease was being found more and more commonly, very focal pockets existed where it was even more common. Just as Snydman had found lots of cases on several country lanes in Connecticut, one of the New York hot spots for Lyme disease was Fire Island. Benach and Hanrahan and the group from Stony Brook began investigating that site. The other site where they were active was on Shelter Island, where Dr. Grunwaldt practiced.

15 • The Culmination of Efforts

As the 1970s merged into the 1980s, at least five groups were hard at work deciphering the riddle of what caused Lyme disease—Steere and the Yale group, Anderson and the team from the CAES, Jorge Benach and the Stony Brook group, and Klaus Weber and Rudolph Ackermann in Germany. Willy Burgdorfer was not directly one of them, but because he was an expert in evaluating ticks, Benach and Grunwaldt sent some Shelter Island ticks to him for analysis in 1981, leading to a major development in the Lyme disease story.

Despite the loss of funding for the study of tick-borne spirochetoses, Burgdorfer had stayed on at the Rocky Mountain Laboratories. There were other tick-borne diseases to study, and Burgdorfer's attention was drawn to them—especially to Colorado tick fever, spread by a virus, and to RMSF. Burgdorfer was now one of the few men in the country, if not the world, who had extensive knowledge and experience in the complex task of evaluating ticks for various pathogens. "Tick surgery is what we do, and what I've done for the last 30 years or so, ever since I got started in this game," Burgdorfer once said. "You take the tick and fix its legs in paraffin on a plate and when the paraffin cools, you take an eye scalpel [the same precision instrument used by eye surgeons] and cut." Just imagine cutting open a tick that's the size of a sesame seed. If that isn't difficult enough, you have to know what's normal and what's abnormal once you're in there.

Burgdorfer had also become an expert on RMSF; in fact, the Rocky Mountain Laboratories had originally been developed to investigate the disease. The revival of interest in tick-borne diseases was stimulating enough for anyone interested in the field. With the arrival of Lyme disease on the landscape, everything shifted. Suddenly, the business of ticks and spirochetes was becoming popular again, with scientists and administrators alike.

But while Burgdorfer's main work was not on Lyme disease, he was not completely out of the loop. As early as the summer of 1977, Steere had telephoned Burgdorfer to solicit his advice about methods of evaluating ticks for pathogenic microorganisms. "In the ensuing lengthy conversation," wrote Burgdorfer, "I emphasized that every tick, regardless of species, carries its own endocytobiotic bacteria, and that a thorough knowledge of the morphology and distribution of these symbiotes is essential before secondarily acquired pathogens can be evaluated. We also discussed the technical aspects of the hemolymph test." Translation: Ticks are very complex creatures that contain many different organisms that naturally occur within them. Only when these are understood, can other, pathogenic organisms be uncovered.

Several weeks later, Steere called Burgdorfer a second time to discuss these complexities further.

In 1978, Burgdorfer spent an eight-month sabbatical with Dr. A. Aeschlimann, director of the Zoological Institute of Neuchâtel, Switzerland. It is perhaps ironic that twenty-seven years after leaving Switzerland, Burgdorfer was once again looking for *C. burnetii*, the rickettsial agent of Q fever, in ticks. And as it had been twenty-seven years previously, the search was once again unsuccessful. This project, however, like the one so many years earlier, also had an unexpected dividend.

As Burgdorfer put it: "Although we failed to find it [*C. burnetii*], we did discover a hitherto undescribed spotted fever rickettsia in up to 11.7% of *I. ricinus,* the most common tick vector in Europe. While dissecting ticks to remove tissues, I noted in the hemocele [a tick's rudimentary blood-filled circulation system] of six ticks, the undulating, waving movements of microfilariae. When isolated and stained, they were identified as the larval stage of *Dipetalonema rugosicauda*, a parasite of deer." They published these findings. When Burgdorfer returned to the United States, he brought with him the stained specimens from 135 *I. ricinus* ticks as reference material. These ticks had been collected in the Seewald Forest on the Swiss plateau, an area of Switzerland where Lyme disease is common.

He returned to the work that he had always been doing, including the project that he and Benach were pursuing with RMSF on Long Island. In the *D. variabilis* ticks, the only organism that the researchers could find was *R. montana*, a nonpathogenic strain of rickettsia. Since they were unable to find the *R. rickettsia* they were looking for in the *D. variabilis* ticks, they figured that they would look in the *I. dammini* because it was possible that this tick was playing a role in the upsurge in RMSF on Long Island. Burgdorfer went through "several hundred of these ticks" using the hemolymph test; all were negative for rickettsia.

Benach had also been working with Edgar Grunwaldt on the babesiosis problem on Shelter Island. Spotted fever was common there, and so was Lyme disease. In fact, the two New York doctors had seen many patients who had both babesiosis and Lyme disease. One other minor clue had led to Benach investigating the *I. dammini* tick. "The spotted fever cases we had," says Benach, "clustered very dramatically in the months of May and June. There were stragglers on either side, but to find one in the fall was peculiar. And in the year 1980, there had been one such case in the fall. And the tick that is active in the fall is the adult *Ixodes dammini*. That gave us the idea that maybe we should look into this because that tick could also be transmitting [RMSF]."

That was late fall 1980, too late to collect many ticks, so they waited until the next season. In October 1981, Benach sent a particular batch of *I. dammini* ticks from Shelter Island to be examined for rickettsiae. Burgdorfer was aware of the context of all these tick-borne illnesses when he performed the hemolymph test on the forty-four male and female ticks. There were no rickettsiae. But two of the female ticks "contained large microfilariae similar to those *(D. rugosicauda)* I had detected three years earlier in the body fluid of the European sheep tick, *I. ricinus*." Burgdorfer then reasoned that for the microfilariae to obtain access to the hemolymph, they must have penetrated the midgut epithelial cells. Out of curiosity, he dissected both of these ticks and made smear preparations from tiny outpouchings in the midgut called diverticula. He stained the preps with Giemsa stain and looked at them using conventional microscopy.

In Burgdorfer's own words: "Instead [of seeing the microfilariae], my attention was captured by faintly stained, rather long and irregularly coiled, individual or clumped microorganisms that looked like spirochetes. Dark-field microscopy of additional diverticulum preparations confirmed their spirochetal nature. Other tissues, including malpighian tubules, central ganglion, ovary, and salivary glands, were free of spirochetes.

"As I watched the rather sluggish slow movements of these organisms, I remembered Hellerstrom's paper and the related discussion presented at the 43rd annual meeting of the Southern Medical Association in Cincinnati, Ohio, in 1949. I could not help but thinking that the microfilariae had led me to the long sought causative agent of ECM and possibly of Lyme disease. Within hours of the discovery, I dissected 124 remaining ticks and examined their tissues microscopically. Seventy-five (60 percent) contained spirochetes that were limited to the midgut."

After so many others had failed, had Willy Burgdorfer discovered the agent that caused Lyme disease?

If he had, he had certainly not proved it, having not even fulfilled the first of Koch's postulates; he hadn't found the presumed agent in a patient with the disease, only in the vector. Burgdorfer, like Koch, was a careful scientist, so he knew that he had a lot more work ahead of him.

He notified Benach immediately. Benach's foresight of maintaining a whole bank of stored convalescent serum samples from Grunwaldt's patients on Shelter Island now paid off. He sent these specimens to Burgdorfer, who made an IFA test to see whether the

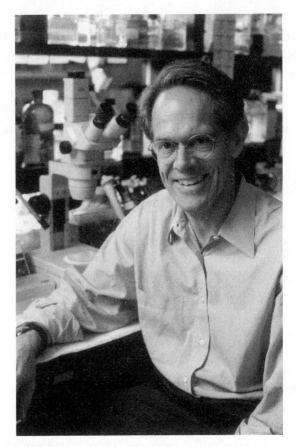

Figure 17. Alan Barbour, M.D., was the first person to grow *Borrelia burgdorferi* on artificial medium and is a world expert on borreliae. (Courtesy of Alan Barbour, M.D.)

antibody from the patients bound to the antigen from their newly discovered spirochete. He also contacted another colleague at the Rocky Mountain Laboratories—Dr. Alan Barbour (Figure 17), a physician and microbiologist who had been working on the relapsing fever borrelia *B. hermsii*. His lab had the capability of culturing borreliae. Barbour had just returned from the Interscience Conference on Antimicrobial Agents and Chemotherapy in Chicago. It was about this time when Steere and Schmid presented data about the new leptospire that they had isolated.

Barbour had learned about cultivating *Borrelia* from Dr. Stoenner, who had developed the method at the Rocky Mountain Laboratories. On November 13, 1981, using Kelly's medium as fortified by Stoenner, Barbour tried to culture the spirochetes. He placed the midgut tissues into capped tubes containing the medium and waited. On November 18, after incubating at thirty-five degrees centigrade for five days, Barbour called Burgdorfer and told him that several of the tubes had spirochetes that could be subcultured. His lab notebook entry read, "Tubes #4, 5, 6 all have spirochetes! Borrelialike." But there was more work ahead for the microbiologist. Two other organisms contaminated the cultures. Barbour labored for another two weeks until he found that by adding certain antibiotics he could suppress the growth of contaminants but not affect the spirochete.

The scientists did three more experiments before making any firm conclusions. They performed the IFA test and found that the serum from Grunwaldt's patients (and a scientist from the State Health Department who had Lyme disease) was strongly positive. Barbour also performed a Western blot test (discussed in Chapter 19) on the serum; the test from the early serum was negative, but a later serum sample was positive. Finally, they tested control sera from patients who never had Lyme disease and found these specimens were uniformly negative.

Recall that in the IFA test, the technician interpreting the test looks for how much of the fluorescein tag is still bound to the antigen and how dilute the serum sample can be and still show fluorescence. When Barbour and Burgdorfer tested these samples, they positively lit up! The lowest titer that they found was 1:80 and the highest was 1:1,280 (Figure 18); that is to say, the levels of antibodies to this new spirochete were astronomical.

But the researchers went further. They allowed infected ticks to feed on laboratory rabbits and found that not only did the rabbits develop ECM-like skin lesions ten to twelve weeks after a tick bite,

Titration of Grosz & Glass sera
versus spirochetes in gut smear of
I. dammini

	1:40	1:80	1:160	1:320	1:640	1:1280
Grosz	###	###	###	###	##	+
Glass	###	##	###	+	+	(+)
NYC 234	—	—	Anti-Human Ig (1:100)			

Grosz : > 1:1280
Glass : 1:640

same - test against rickettsia-like agent

	1:40	1:80	1:160	1:320	
Grosz	+ to ##	(+)	(+)	(+)	a few coccal org. stain
Glass	##	+	(+)	(+)	occasional reaction weak
NYC 234	—			Anti-Human Ig 1:100	

occasional st. of bac. ... very weak

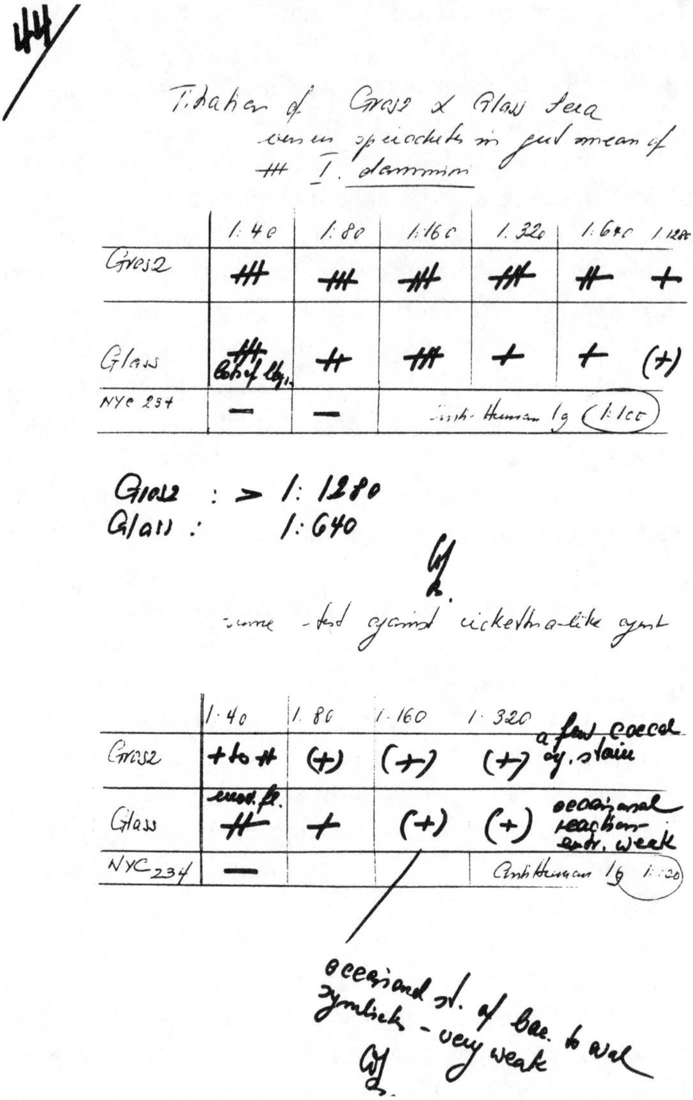

Figure 18. Willy Burgdorfer's results of an indirect immunofluoresence test (December 29, 1981) with sera of two patients recovered from Lyme arthritis. Both had high titers (up to 1:1,280) and reacted strongly with spirochetes on preparations from tick midgut tissues or cultures. They were negative when treated with a nonspecific conjugate (against rickettsiae) or with sera from healthy people. (Courtesy of Willy Burgdorfer)

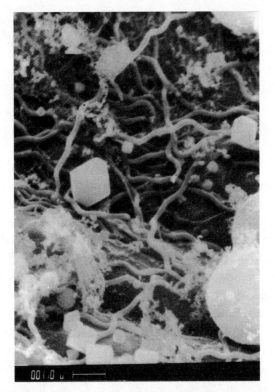

Figure 19. Scanning electron micrograph of *Borrelia burgdorferi* in the gut of an *Ixodes scapularis* tick from Shelter Island, New York. Bar = 1.0 micron. (Photograph courtesy of Stanley F. Hayes, Dan Dorward, and Willy Burgdorfer, Rocky Mountain Laboratories, Hamilton, Montana.)

but also the rabbits' serum reacted strongly to the *I. dammini* spirochete, as it was called at this point.

In June 1982, Burgdorfer, along with several other colleagues, including Barbour, Benach, and Grunwaldt, published their findings in *Science*. This initial strain of bacteria was referred to as the B31 strain, so named because it was the first isolate of the three Bs— Burgdorfer, Benach, and Barbour (Figure 19).

This finding and publication refocused the work of almost all of the other groups that had been searching for the agent of Lyme

disease. Within one year, each of them had produced significant findings. In the March 31, 1983, issue of the *New England Journal of Medicine,* two reports appeared showing isolation of the new *I. dammini*
spirochete in patients with Lyme disease. Steere and colleagues and
Benach and colleagues each reported isolating the new organism. The
Yale group found the spirochete in three of fifty-six patients studied,
isolating the new organism in the blood of one patient, the skin of
another, and the cerebrospinal fluid of the third. The Stony Brook
team found the organism in the blood of two of their thirty-six patients. In this paper Benach noted that three of the four Koch's postulates had been "largely satisfied": "the organism has been isolated
from patients with Lyme disease (although not all patients), it has
been cultured [on artificial medium], and it can be used to induce
an ECM-like lesion in rabbits." The only link in Koch's chain of
causality not yet accomplished was isolating the spirochete from the
experimental animals, the rabbits, after they had been experimentally infected. Burgdorfer and his colleagues unsuccessfully attempted
this.

In Germany, Dr. Weber probably spoke for many people in the
field when he said: "The discovery meant a shock and relief all together for me: a shock because we had wasted so much time to discover the organism and relief that all was over now. All I could do
was to congratulate Willy and his group."

But the investigators still did not know a lot about this new
organism. Initially, they were not even clear whether it was a treponeme
or a borrelia; everyone was still using the term "*I. dammini* spirochete."
So investigation continued. Now that the organism was found, teams
using the IFA test could test serum samples that they had stored in freez-
ers for the past decade. Ackermann and colleagues found a spirochete
in the bloodstream of a woman with ECM and found antibodies to a
spirochete closely related to *B. duttoni* in half of their patients with ECM
and 90 percent of their patients with neurological symptoms. Similarly,
Swedish doctors from the Karolinksa Institute and Lund University also
found that their patients with neurological syndromes related to Lyme
disease had antibodies to this new, still unnamed spirochete.

Burgdorfer and Barbour were instrumental in many of these discoveries and were the first to report the spirochete in the European *I. ricinus* tick as well. While Barbour went to work on culturing the spirochetes, Burgdorfer continued his work, too. Within days of his original discovery, he had also found these spirochetes in *I. ricinus*. "During my sabbatical in 1978, I had prepared hundreds of smears of tissues during tick/rickettsial surveys on the Swiss Plateau," recalls Burgdorfer. "Several boxes had been brought back to the United States as reference material. Slides still available were stained by Giemsa and reexamined. Spirochetes similar to those in *I. dammini* were found in 13 (17 percent) of 135 smears."

While these studies were being undertaken, the group from the Rocky Mountain Laboratories asked for and was granted permission to import live *I. ricinus* ticks from Europe. They received about six hundred ticks, dissected them, and found that one-third of them had spirochetes, which under the microscope closely resembled their New World counterparts. Burgdorfer next turned his attention to the *I. pacificus* tick, the vector of those cases of Lyme disease that were being reported in the Pacific Northwest. In these ticks, too, though only in a small percentage, he found spirochetes that were visually indistinguishable from those in *I. dammini* and *I. ricinus*.

Also in 1983, Anderson and Magnarelli from the CAES published their results of finding the spirochetes in the midgut of the ticks that they had pulled off the mice and raccoons from the Lyme and East Haddam sites they had been investigating. They also found the spirochete in the blood from some of the rodents. On further testing, they found the spirochetes to be both morphologically and serologically the same as the Shelter Island (B31) strain; that is to say, they looked the same under the microscope, and they reacted to the same antibodies from the serum as the spirochetes that Burgdorfer, Benach, and Barbour had reported.

Much of this work was done simultaneously. While Burgdorfer's work crystallized that of the other teams, each group had been pursuing similar lines of investigation. Thus, 1982 and 1983 were seminal years in the history of Lyme disease. Work reported in these years was the culmination of the efforts of hundreds of scientists and doctors. All had put an enormous effort toward discovering the mysteries of Lyme disease since at least 1975—even longer in the case of the European researchers such as Weber and Ackermann. Finally, a specific spirochete had been identified in the tick vector, in the animal reservoirs, and in some human patients with Lyme disease. Also in 1983, the Lyme disease spirochete would be given its official name.

16 • Progress to the End of the 1980s

The "coming-out" party of Lyme disease occurred in November 1983, when the First International Symposium on Lyme Disease was held in New Haven. As Allen Steere wrote in the preface to the publication of the proceedings from that conference: "When Lyme disease was described eight years ago, we hoped that someday it would be an established entity, that multiple investigators would be working on the problem, and that we would meet to discuss our work. The First International Symposium on Lyme Disease is a dream come true. Lyme disease has come of age."

Participants and contributors from thirteen states and four countries traveled to New Haven to mark the occasion. They presented data from their own work and experiences and listened to the experiences of others. Some were medical doctors, others were Ph.D.s, and still others were doctors of public health. There were rheumatologists, neurologists, entomologists, infectious diseases specialists, dermatologists, and many others.

Polly Murray also attended. She remembered how different if felt for her to be driving down to Yale for this symposium compared with her first visits to the medical library nearly ten years before when she had been researching her own baffling array of symptoms. Mrs. Murray met with and spoke to many of the researchers, such as Klaus Weber, Andrew Spielman, John Anderson, and Louis Magnarelli. At one point, she addressed the assembly to communicate the perspective of a patient. She emphasized the importance of public education initiatives and what doctors refer to as "soft" symptoms—that is, the psychological signs such as depression and mood and behavioral problems. She also spoke about organizing patient support groups. After her remarks, she recalls Dr. Malawista saying, "Knowing Mrs. Murray's track record, all of these things may very well get done over the next [few] years."

The scientists summarized their years of work. Steere and his group described many clinical manifestations that had never been reported in Europe. Other researchers detailed the relationship between Lyme disease and the tick vectors in the *Ixodes* genus (*dammini, ricinus,* and *pacificus*). The basic scientists discussed the structure and immunology of the germ. But it was also at this conference that a name for the spirochete, now determined to be a borrelia, was announced: *Borrelia burgdorferi,* honoring Willy Burgdorfer.

Since Burgdorfer's discovery in 1981, the bug had been referred to as the "*I. dammini* spirochete" or the "Lyme disease spirochete." This is akin to a hospital identifying a newborn as "baby boy Jones" until the parents name their new son. But "baby boy Jones" would no better do as a permanent name for a child than the "Lyme disease spirochete" would for a microorganism. Russ Johnson, a microbiologist from the University of Minnesota who was one of the lead researchers of the spirochete, called an informal meeting to discuss the official name, much like a judge might initiate a sidebar conversation with lawyers in a trial to clarify a point of law. This was an unusual step. Normally, the scientist who was publishing the scientific paper describing the organism would name it. Because the precise nature of the spirochete was not clear at the time of the original discovery of Burgdorfer and colleagues, Johnson did the subsequent work. And he had the wisdom to get buy-in from the various stakeholders first.

In the room were Steere, Johnson, Weber, Barbour, Benach,

Burgdorfer, and several others. As the genus of the organism was known, the first part of the name would be *Borrelia*. The question before the group was what should follow that—the species name. Some argued that the species name should reflect the biological tendencies of the organism, such as *Borrelia rheumatica*. Other possibilities could mark the location of the U.S. outbreak, such as *Borrelia lymeii*. And another possibility was to honor one of the scientists involved in its discovery. Although the scientists in the room did not uniformly agree, they eventually decided, and the organism was officially designated *Borrelia burgdorferi*.

Also at the conference, the European doctors presented their perspective, dominating the sessions on the neurological manifestations of Lyme disease. Just as the joint manifestations of Lyme disease seemed to be far more common in the United States, the neurological symptoms were being reported more frequently in Germany and Scandinavia. In addition, there were talks on the distribution of Lyme disease—from various parts of the United States other than the East Coast, such as Wisconsin and Minnesota, to its global distribution.

By the middle to late 1980s, textbooks would have told you that Lyme disease was caused by infection with the spirochete *B. burgdorferi*, which was transmitted by the bite of an infected *Ixodes* tick, *I. dammini*, in much of North America and the bite of other species in other parts of the world. Some patients would not get sick after such a tick bite; others would. For those who fell ill, the majority would develop an unusual skin rash called erythema migrans that would usually begin roughly seven to ten days after the tick bite. The rash was flat and red, often had central clearing, and could grow to large sizes. This was the first stage of the disease.

If the patient remained untreated, the rash would ultimately resolve. Some patients would never develop further symptoms, presumably because the microscopic battle between their immune system and the spirochete's invasive arsenal ended in favor of the patient. About 15 percent of the patients, however, would develop stage two symptoms over the ensuing weeks to months. These included neurological problems, such as a cranial nerve infection like Bell's palsy, or a mild form of meningitis or the same radiculitis that Garin and Buja-doux first reported. A bit less than 10 percent of these untreated patients would show signs of inflammation of their hearts. Some would exhibit an electrical malfunction of their hearts, resulting in dangerously slow pulses.

Months to years after the initial tick bite, about 60 percent of untreated patients would develop arthritis, often of the knee, swelling to grotesque proportions. Still others began having funny sensations in their limbs from neuropathy, while other patients became forgetful and unable to sleep or think normally, a condition called encephalopathy. The Yale group showed that oral antibiotic therapy was useful for stage one symptoms and that intravenous penicillin was of value for the later stage two and stage three symptoms.

Regarding the arthritis, Malawista gave a presentation at the First International Symposium about how Lyme disease was, as he had predicted in 1976, a unique model for other forms of arthritis. Having a form of arthritis where the "zero time" was known was, Malawista noted, "the stuff that rheumatologists' dreams are made of"; that is, because Lyme arthritis had a definable onset, marked by the rash, rheumatologists could study the joint inflammation in a way that they could not for, say, rheumatoid arthritis or lupus.

Even as early as 1983, however, as Dr. Steere summarized at the symposium, differences had been highlighted between Lyme disease seen in the United States and that seen in Europe. "Both arthritis and carditis following EM have now been described in Europe, but they are rare," he wrote. "Conversely, two additional entities—lymphocytoma and acrodermatitis chronica atrophicans [ACA]—have been linked to EM and *Ixodes ricinus* tick bites in Europe, but an association with tick bites has not been recognized in the United States. In general, the disease seems more virulent in America—multiple skin lesions are more common, headache occurs more often with the meningitis, and arthritis is a frequent feature of the disease—but the basic outlines of the illness are similar both here and abroad."

The cause of Lyme disease was now well-established, and the need for antibiotic treatment had been shown beyond the shadow of a doubt. After all the research and with all of this information, why didn't Lyme disease go the way of toxic shock syndrome and Legionnaire's disease—that is, why did Lyme disease continue to grow, on both geographical and sociopolitical levels? Both toxic shock syndrome and Legionnaire's disease in the late 1970s had made big media splashes. In fact, both were in some important ways even more alarming than Lyme disease because both were associated with significant mortality. Twenty-nine of the original legionnaires in the Philadelphia outbreak died from the pneumonia. Toxic shock syndrome had killed healthy young women. But after a few years, articles in the lay press about these diseases disappeared; they no longer graced the covers of national news magazines. And also unlike Lyme disease, dozens of patient support groups and Internet sites did not spring up for these diseases; nor were they the subject of U.S. Senate hearings (see Chapter 25).

Why did Lyme disease continue to grow? This question is best split into two: "Why did the incidence and geographical range of Lyme disease continue to expand?" and "Why did public concern and the sociopolitical profile of Lyme disease increase?" But first, we must address two points of nomenclature.

Recall that Andrew Spielman believed that the tick originally called *Ixodes scapularis* was in fact a new species, which he named *Ixodes dammini*. This change (from *scapularis* to *dammini*) was not to stand. In 1993, Dr. James Oliver, a professor of entomology at Georgia Southern University, and colleagues published a paper detailing evidence that *I. scapularis* and *I. dammini* were, in fact, identical and not two separate species. Many of the experiments he and his colleagues performed showed that ticks from both regions of the United States (the Northeast and the Southeast) would mate and produce progeny. He therefore proposed that since the name *I. scapularis* had priority, it should be the formal scientific name of the black-legged tick, sometimes referred to as the deer tick. Spielman still disputes the name change.

Lest the reader think such disputes are a matter of the modern ego, nearly one hundred years ago a nearly identical argument occurred regarding the naming of the tick *D. andersoni*, the agent of RMSF in the western states. In 1904, Dr. Charles Stiles, a U.S. public health physician, named the tick *D. reticulatus*. He later changed his mind, thinking that while these ticks were closely related to *D. reticulatus*, they were sufficiently different to warrant a new species name. The following year, he wrote a paper and referred to the tick as *D. andersoni*, in honor of the physician John F. Anderson. Then in 1906, Howard Ricketts and W. W. King both reported that *D. occidentalis* was the vector of RMSF.

Then another entomologist, Nathan Banks, entered the fray, referring to the tick as *D. venustus*. Stiles almost immediately rejected this notion, and the two men jousted in letters to the editor in *JAMA*, in which Banks accused Stiles of a "gross violation of the rules of nomenclature." The issue was not resolved until 1924, when the International Commission on Zoological Nomenclature voted to officially name the tick *D. andersoni*. Thus, this kind of dispute in nomenclature is by no means new. Even at the time that Stiles was embroiled in his dispute, he wrote in 1910 that the confusion over *D. andersoni* "has simply repeated the history of many other species."

The effect of a seemingly innocuous change in nomenclature can be more important than the initial superficial disagreement—as was the case with Lyme disease. The range of *I. dammini* was limited to the northeastern United States, but *I. scapularis* could be found across the southeast and southern states as well. Having a known vector for *B. burgdorferi* in other areas of the country opened the possibility that Lyme disease might occur elsewhere than in the Northeast. Therefore, the deer tick was initially referred to as *I. scapularis* until 1979 when Spielman published his paper suggesting a new species, *I. dammini*. Then beginning in 1993, the name flipped back to *I. scapularis*, as we will do now for the remainder of this story.

Another name change occurred at about this same time. The acronym ECM, for erythema chronicum migrans, yielded to EM, for erythema migrans. Back in 1913 Lipschutz had used the term ECM and had failed to reference the prior name, EM, that Afzelius had given the rash three years before. Klaus Weber in 1986 argued that the term EM was older (and thus had priority), more descriptive (because many cases were not so chronic—hence the *chronicum* in ECM), and simpler. This shift also occurred in the medical literature, although it was associated with a great deal less emotion, probably because the name of a living person was not in jeopardy.

Despite all the questions that had been answered into the 1980s, two still occupied both the public and scientists: Why did Lyme disease continue to become increasingly common? and, How long had it existed? Recall that for decades doctors in the area of Montauk Point, Long Island, had talked of "Montauk knee" and "Montauk spider bite." At the time, these were thought to represent conditions whose causes were unknown, but in retrospect, they were almost certainly due to Lyme disease. The same phenomenon occurred in other areas. For instance, on Cape Cod, Massachusetts, the first case of Lyme disease occurred in 1962—diagnosed retrospectively, that is, years after the patient's symptoms, after the concept of Lyme disease emerged.

How much farther back in time did Lyme disease occur? In Europe, the first case of what we now know to be part of the spectrum of diseases caused by *B. burgdorferi* was reported in 1883 (the case of ACA reported by Buchwald). Did immigrants to the United States from the Old World import Lyme disease? Some evidence helps to answer this question—evidence from a recent scientific technique called polymerase chain reaction, or PCR.

The genetic code of all living organisms—bacteria, plants, animals, and humans—is composed of deoxyribonucleic acid, or DNA. Our DNA contains the blueprints for everything that we are—the color of our skin, the diseases we acquire—and, if you happen to be a bacterium, the antibiotics that you can defend against, or the form and texture of the proteins on your outer membrane. DNA is a molecule made up of thousands of base pairs—paired groupings of four chemicals called *nucleotides.* These paired nucleotides form a twisted helix that stretches on and on. The DNA of a borrelia is different from the DNA of a treponeme or a leptospire, although the

DNA of these three kinds of spirochete share many more similarities than with the DNA of an orangutan, for instance. Still, differences in the sequences of base pairs do exist between different bacterial species.

In 1983 a biochemist named Kary Mullis conceived of a method for isolating and then reproducing in large quantity small sequences of DNA that make each organism distinct. His method would find a particular strand, or segment, of DNA that, for example, is found only on *B. burgdorferi* and no other organism on the planet and then reproduce that minute segment repeatedly until it reached a measurable quantity. Within a few years, this technique, the PCR, was perfected, and medical diagnostics was revolutionized. DNA testing began to permeate our society—from paternity suits to murder trials to medical diagnostic testing.

One medical researcher who was quick to apply this technique in the medical arena was Dr. David Persing, then at the Yale University Department of Pathology. Being at Yale, Persing was interested in Lyme disease. Among many other projects, he and colleagues used PCR on 102 dried-out or alcohol-preserved tick specimens from the Museum of Comparative Zoology in Cambridge, Massachusetts. The ticks had been collected from various areas in New England between 1945 and 1951; each was tagged with the exact location where they had been collected. The researchers also examined another batch of ticks from the Smithsonian collection in Washington, D.C., some dating back as far as 1924. They found ticks that were positive for the DNA of *B. burgdorferi* from Montauk Point and from the adjacent Heather Hills State Park from the mid-1940s.

Several years later, the same group with additional colleagues reported the results of similar experiments done on tiny biopsy specimens taken from the ears of archived mice from the same museum. They found two specimens that tested positive by PCR analysis for *B. burgdorferi* from mice originally captured near Dennis, Massachusetts (on Cape Cod), in 1894! The DNA from these specimens was identical to the B31 strain that Willy Burgdorfer had found on Shelter Island.

European investigators have reproduced these experiments using archived ticks from various parts of Europe including England and have found borrelial DNA dating back to the late 1880s as well. If the Lyme spirochete had been around for so long, why did it begin to surface as a recognized medical entity only in the past few decades? This question can be answered in one word—deer.

17 • A Geographical Expansion

When the first European settlers arrived in the Northeast, they found land that was described as "park-like." The native inhabitants had maintained this state for a variety of reasons. They used fire to burn the thicket and stimulate the subsequent growth of grass, which served as food for the grazing animals that they hunted. They also required huge amounts of wood to stoke the fires that cooked their food and kept them warm throughout the long New England winters.

Like the native North Americans, the European settlers also used enormous quantities of wood for shelter, heat, and cooking fuel. A single house required approximately twenty cords of wood per year for heating by open fireplaces. The metal tools colonists used allowed them to be even more efficient at chopping down trees. Furthermore, they were farmers, and farms required large tracts of cleared land to provide adequate space for crops. Wood was also converted into charcoal for use in smelting iron and manufacturing glass.

Deer require adequate forest structure both for nourishment and for protection against predators. As the human population grew, the human need for increased farming and for wood for heat, shelter, and cooking grew proportionately. By the 1800s, as a result of deforestation, the deer habitat decreased drastically, as did their numbers.

The island of Martha's Vineyard was virtually stripped of trees during that century. In Concord, Massachusetts, deer were so rare that in 1854, Henry David Thoreau wrote about the lack of deer in the Walden Pond area.

The building of the Erie Canal and the development of the railroads opened the vast expanses of fertile farmland in the Midwest. Grain and cattle could be produced more economically in the Midwest and shipped back to the growing population on the East Coast. The relatively hilly and rocky soil of the Northeast was no longer needed. Farms were much more efficient in the Midwest, and the cheap transportation east by rail resulted in many New England farms being abandoned.

Although we tend to think of our land as being increasingly commercialized and less wooded now compared with a century ago, this is actually not the case. The state of Connecticut, for example, is much more covered with forest now than it was one hundred years ago. In 1860, only 27 percent of that state's land was forested. By 1910, 45 percent was covered by forest, and by 1965, the number rose to 63 percent.

But although the deer habitat and deer were returning, wolves that once roamed freely in the Northeast had been hunted out of existence. It doesn't take an expert in population dynamics to predict the result of such a situation. The deer herd has steadily increased. In Connecticut, the deer herd was estimated at about four thousand in 1936. Twenty years later, it had tripled to twelve thousand. Another twenty years later, in 1976, it had grown to nearly thirty thousand, and in 1996, it exceeded fifty-two thousand.

The adult deer tick's preferred host for spending the winter and mating is the deer. Thus, this increase in the deer herd led to a corresponding increase in the tick population. In the first meeting between Allen Steere and Judith Mensch, Mrs. Mensch had remarked about how common the ticks had become near her home in Old Lyme and wondered aloud whether they might be part of the problem.

Another change in population dynamics is on the human side of the equation. Suburban tracts of land for homes became increasingly popular. So the larger numbers of deer were living closer to humans.

In many areas, people see deer in their yards and neighborhoods every day.

Another component of the formula—the white-footed mouse—is also found in great quantities in these forested areas, especially along the so-called edge zones. These areas were the perfect spot for homes—a picturesque area surrounded by a few low-lying stone walls, shrubs, and bushes, followed by taller trees farther out on the periphery—very similar to the area where the Murray family had their home in Old Lyme.

A similar story has occurred in Europe, where during the Second World War, ancient Old World forests were decimated by bombing and by the need for wood, both as building material for the war effort and as a source of precious fuel for heating and cooking. Deer populations decreased, not only from the destruction of their forested habitat, but also because they were hunted for food during a time when that resource, too, was scarce. Wood also fueled the rapid rebuilding that followed the war. But as European politics stabilized, so did the landscape, and many European forested areas began to return. The deer herd rebounded; human population shifts such as those in the United States occurred, and Lyme disease became increasingly common in Europe as well.

In the United States, the numbers of cases of Lyme disease steadily grew through the 1980s and into the 1990s. In the early 1980s, the number of cases ranged between 500 and 2,500 per year. In 1988, that number rose to nearly 5,000, and in 1989, the national number was 8,803. In 1994, the number of cases broke the 10,000 mark, and in 1998, 16,801 cases were reported to the CDC. Some of this increase reflects changes in reporting regulations. For example, even in Connecticut, Lyme disease became a reportable disease only in 1987, and it became a nationally reportable disease in 1991. Some of this rise in the number of Lyme disease cases is undoubtedly due to heightened recognition by physicians and patients alike. Another factor that is possibly related to the higher numbers is the increase in the availability of blood testing for Lyme disease. Some of this increase, however, almost certainly reflects a true rise in the incidence of the disease.

In addition, there is general agreement that the number of

reported cases is but a fraction of the number of true cases. Many diseases are "reportable" to local health authorities—diseases such as bacterial meningitis, tuberculosis, and sexually transmitted diseases. Generally, doctors are careful to report such diseases because of their obvious public health implications. Alerting public health authorities of cases of meningitis or tuberculosis could prevent the next case and possibly save a life. Unfortunately, doctors are not so compulsive about reporting other diseases, with less obvious, or at least less urgent, public health implications.

In Connecticut, a study undertaken by the state's department of public health surveyed hundreds of physicians in that state who were in a likely position to see Lyme disease—internists, family practitioners, pediatricians, and dermatologists—and found that only 7 percent of them ever reported a single case of Lyme disease during the study year of 1992. These researchers estimated that at best, only 16 percent of Connecticut cases of Lyme disease were being reported. When they extrapolated the data to all of the doctors in the state, they estimated that only 11 percent of Lyme disease cases were being properly reported to the state.

In Maryland, a different team of researchers performed a similar study and got nearly identical results. They concluded that approximately ten times more cases of Lyme disease were treated in that state than reported. Both of these studies were comparing the number of cases diagnosed with the number reported. Lyme disease is fairly common in both of these states. It is possible that in states where Lyme disease is less common, and there is less public knowledge and concern, that even more cases go undiagnosed and even fewer cases are reported.

In the short term, the importance of complete and accurate reporting of Lyme disease (assuming a correct diagnosis) has little immediate effect on the public health, that is, on preventing the next case. Knowing the true amount of Lyme disease cases, however, does help to direct research funding and educational efforts aimed at both doctor and patient. The better the education, the more cases of Lyme disease will be diagnosed early, when prompt treatment has an excellent chance of a cure.

The bottom line is that the true number of cases of Lyme disease may be ten times what the CDC currently reports. This means that, for instance, in 2000, when 18,000 cases were reported to the CDC, 180,000 people may actually have contracted the disease.

Another phenomenon that was playing out in parallel with the numerical increase in the incidence of Lyme disease was the expansion of its geographical range. Early on in the United States it was clear that the disease was found mostly in three pockets—the northeastern states, the north central states, and the Pacific Northwest. Over the next decade, however, Lyme disease was being diagnosed outside these pockets—sometimes in areas where the disease was previously unknown. Was it really Lyme disease? And if so, how was it getting there?

One can use different degrees of scrutiny when looking for anything, and diseases are no exception. Either one can actively search for the disease, called *active surveillance,* or one can sit back and wait for reports of it to come in, called *passive surveillance.* One of the first physicians to begin organized active surveillance was George Schmid of the CDC. In 1984, he and colleagues from state health departments in Minnesota and Wisconsin, as well as Yale and the CDC, tabulated Lyme disease cases that had been reported in 1982. They found the same three familiar pockets of Lyme but also noted that cases were appearing sporadically in states nonendemic for the disease. They divided their cases into "definite" and "probable."

An *endemic area* refers to one in which a given disease occurs regularly. In Schmid's study, an endemic area was considered a county located two or fewer counties away from one that had previously reported a definite case of the disease. The definition of "definite" was based on clinical manifestations in an endemic area. If a case exhibited no EM, it was defined as a probable case. This is a bit circular, as the two variables (endemic or nonendemic, and definite versus probable) were not independent and in fact were closely related. But these were the earliest days of Lyme disease surveillance, and the investigators had to start somewhere.

The sporadic cases (all of which Schmid and colleagues defined as probable, not definite) had been reported in Kentucky, Indiana, and Montana. Were these reports justified? Was this really Lyme disease, or simply diagnostic error?

In areas where Lyme disease was already endemic, its range was clearly expanding. At the outset of the Connecticut outbreak, Lyme disease had been far more common on the eastern shore of the Connecticut River compared with the western. But over the years, active surveillance showed that the western shore was catching up.

Using active surveillance, researchers noted and described a focal epidemic of Lyme disease in coastal Massachusetts, in the town of Ipswich. During the mid-1970s the white-tailed deer had become quite common in the area of a nature preserve. The preserve bordered a barrier beach area on one side. An access road led into the protected area, and about 200 year-round residents lived in the 160 or so homes situated along that road. The researchers collected blood samples and administered health questionnaires. Over seven years, more than one-third of the 190 residents studied contracted Lyme disease.

In New York, the state health department also engaged in active surveillance of Lyme disease, studying both the case reports of the disease and ticks collected from birds, rodents, and deer. The number of cases of Lyme disease reported in 1982 was 106, and in 1989 it rose to 1,942 cases. Some of this increase may have been due to the fact that reporting guidelines changed over those years, becoming mandatory rather than voluntary. Some of it may also have been because over that period of time in New York both patients and doctors had become more aware of Lyme disease. But the researchers concluded that the number of cases had truly risen. More interesting, however, was that they found that the *number* of counties reporting Lyme disease had clearly increased. This expansion was mirrored in the tick studies. *Ixodes scapularis* ticks were being found in areas where previously they had not been. This led additional support to their conclusion that the increases in human cases were not simply a function of the change in reporting regulations or better recognition by physicians and patients.

Scientists speculated that birds were spreading the ticks. Expansion of the number and range of deer herds could certainly account for some of the geographical expansion of Lyme disease, but not all of it. Increases in the range of deer would allow for a gradual expansion of the current boundaries of the ticks, but not the rapid increases that physicians and epidemiologists were now tracking. Ticks hitching rides on birds, however, would account for a more rapid and wider-ranging increase in the range of the disease.

Anderson and Magnarelli knew that ticks would parasitize various species of birds, but scientists from the University of Maine, led by Robert Smith, showed conclusively that migrating birds could facilitate the long-distance dispersal of *I. scapularis*. They did this by showing that infected ticks hitched rides on birds to an island off the southern coast of Maine, on which Lyme disease had not occurred. Two ornithologists on the team were working on a bird-banding project on Appledore Island, one of the Isles of Shoals archipelago. While banding thousands of birds, they would search the birds' heads and necks for ticks, removing any that they found for later identification by a trained entomologist. They found that infected ticks did hitch rides on migratory birds, and also that the genetic analysis of the *B. burgdorferi* in these ticks was identical to the common strains found along the nearby coast.

Although having infected ticks from an endemic area drop off in a nonendemic area is necessary for establishing a new focus of Lyme disease, it is not sufficient. The ticks would also need to find a competent host, such as the white-footed mouse, and there must be deer or another large mammal on which the adult ticks will mate and spend the winter. The mouse or other host would be necessary for maintaining a reservoir to infect new ticks. The deer or other large mammal would be necessary for the adult ticks to complete their part of the life cycle. Nevertheless, the findings by Smith and his colleagues opened the possibility that birds were spreading Lyme disease to new areas.

One new area where Lyme disease seemed to be turning up was Georgia, although just looking at the numbers, one would not think there was a problem. During 1989, physicians from that state reported 715 cases of the disease to the CDC; but in 1990, they reported 161 cases and only 28 in 1991. These physicians were seeing the rash of EM, so they reported Lyme disease. The CDC, however, told them

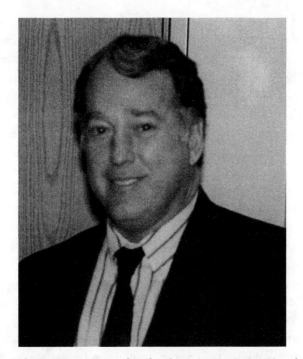

Figure 20. Ed Masters, M.D., a family physician in Cape Girardeau, Missouri, has unsuccessfully tried to persuade the Centers for Disease Control and Prevention that his patients have Lyme disease. The CDC does not consider Missouri to be endemic area. (Courtesy of Ed Masters, M.D.)

that there was no documented cycle in nature of *B. burgdorferi* in Georgia so Lyme disease could not exist there. The physicians stopped reporting it. What happened in that state? According to James Oliver, the tick expert responsible for the name change from *dammini* back to *scapularis,* the situation in the South is more complex than that in the Northeast and other areas of the country. There seems to be more biological diversity in the spirochetes that are found as well as the tick vectors and animal reservoirs. Something seemed to be causing Lyme disease in Georgia, but whatever it was, it was invisible to the CDC.

A similar story played out in Missouri. Ed Masters (Figure 20), a family physician in Cape Girardeau, Missouri, has found himself embroiled in this controversy over the geographical bounds of Lyme disease. Masters tells the story of how he got involved in Lyme disease as follows: "My avocation is tree forestry. I've always been interested in it and belonged to some forestry organizations, and in fact one of my passions is I like to plant walnut trees. In 1987, I was on the executive committee of the national walnut council and we were planning our next meeting, which was going to be held in Wisconsin, and the president said 'You know Ed, a lot of our members, especially in the north and out East, are getting concerned about Lyme disease. And I think we owe it to our members to give them an update on Lyme disease, and you're a doctor so why don't you do it?' I just looked at him and laughed and said, 'Lyme disease, you must be joking.' I said we didn't even know about it when I was in medical school, and I said furthermore it doesn't even exist in Missouri."

Masters nonetheless was successfully corralled into giving the lecture. Being a man who does not do something halfway, he began to research the subject prodigiously. During the six months that he was preparing the lecture, he noticed that some of his patients had rashes that looked like the ones in the pictures he was seeing in articles about Lyme disease. He reported four cases to the state board of health. However, he says: "The first four cases were thrown out of the state computer without so much as a courtesy [of a phone call]. They were just removed. I've been in practice for about twenty-two years. It's not like I'm a spring chicken or anything. And I was not known for making radical statements that I can't back up. In fact, I had a closed practice at the time. I wasn't even taking new patients; I didn't need the patients; I didn't need the controversy."

But Masters is also not one to back off when controversy finds him. He was seeing patients whose rashes looked exactly like EM. He would biopsy the rash and show them to pathologists, who agreed that they were consistent with EM. He treated the patients with antibiotics, and the rashes would rapidly resolve. Furthermore, he saw patients with other Lyme-related conditions, such as Bell's palsy and heart conduction problems. According to Masters, "If it looks like a duck, walks like a duck, and quacks like a duck, there's a good chance it is a duck." He continued to diagnose Lyme disease, but he took some additional steps that most practicing clinicians would not have taken.

He began storing patients' serum samples in a freezer and performing skin biopsies of the rashes to culture the specimens. He sent them to various pathologists around the country. He also began linking up with scientists from across the country to sort out exactly what the phenomenon was that he was seeing. He tried and tried to culture *B. burgdorferi* from his patients but was unsuccessful. Dr. Oliver from Georgia was one of the scientists Masters had contacted, but they could not find *B. burgdorferi* in the patient specimens from Missouri.

Many of Masters's patients remembered being bitten by a tick that had a big white spot on its back—a tick that could only be the Lone Star tick, or *Amblyomma americanum*. Because this was not the classic vector for Lyme disease, and because *B. burgdorferi* could not be cultured from either the patients or the ticks, the CDC refused to acknowledge that Missouri harbored Lyme disease. But Masters persisted.

The difficulty in proving geographical expansion of Lyme disease to areas outside of the usual locations was not just a problem with the tick vectors. It also got to the heart of how doctors diagnosed Lyme disease. The CDC definition for diagnosis of early Lyme disease was "physician-diagnosed EM that is greater than five centimeters [about two and one half inches] in size." In these early cases, blood testing was not a part of the case-finding definition. So using the CDC's own definition, physicians in Georgia and Missouri reported that they were seeing Lyme disease. But because the cases were in a nonendemic area, the CDC tossed out these purely clinical diagnoses.

The diagnosis of later stages of Lyme disease would require laboratory confirmation, but if there were problems in defining the expanding geography of Lyme disease, there were even bigger problems with the blood tests.

18 • The Diagnostician's Dilemma

To fully understand why Lyme disease has become controversial and such a lightning rod of public concern, one must understand the diagnostic problems associated with how Lyme disease—or any disease—is diagnosed.

Some diagnoses are obvious: A patient arrives at the emergency department with an arrow sticking out beneath his right third rib. He is diagnosed as having a penetrating injury to the chest. The doctor may not know which organs have been damaged, but she does know that an arrow is sticking out of the patient's chest. There is nothing subtle or ambiguous about this situation.

This is sometimes the case with Lyme disease. A patient visits her doctor's office in July with a rash. She has spent a considerable amount of time outdoors along the Connecticut shore. She pulled an engorged deer tick off her right side, just below her right third rib, a week before. She now feels some mild muscle aches and has a low-grade fever and notices a round, flat, red rash on her torso where the tick bit her. The rash does not hurt or itch, and over the two days since the bite, it has gradually expanded and is now about six inches in diameter. This is the Lyme disease equivalent of having an arrow sticking out of the chest. No blood test, biopsy, or any other test is necessary for a clear diagnosis.

Unfortunately, there is often considerably more uncertainty in diagnosis than a patient with classic EM after a tick bite. In such cases, doctors often perform laboratory tests to help them increase or decrease their confidence in a diagnosis. But these tests are rarely black-or-white indicators of health versus disease. You may see such clarity on television medical shows, but that is because one-hour programs do not lend themselves to real-life diagnostic ambiguity.

But if tests are not 100 percent accurate, how is their accuracy measured? How do doctors know how to incorporate these results into real-life clinical decision making if the answers are not black or white? Accuracy of diagnostic tests is typically discussed in terms of their *sensitivity* and *specificity*. A test can be very sensitive (it will be positive, or abnormal, in patients with the disease) and very specific (it will be negative, or normal, in patients without the disease). A test that is very sensitive is good at identifying true-positives. A test that is very specific is good at identifying true-negatives; which is to say, there will be few false-positives. A test that is 95 percent sensitive and 95 percent specific is an excellent test for physicians—not perfect, but very good and in keeping with many tests used every day in medicine. Some of the best Lyme disease blood tests are about this accurate, and few tests in medicine are much better.

However, a test that is both 95 percent sensitive and specific will lead to incorrect information some of the time. How good that test is at identifying patients with a given disease will in part depend on which patients are being tested. To better understand this concept, let us temporarily step away from medicine and consider an example that is simultaneously abstract and concrete—a test that distinguishes peaches from other types of fruit.

Imagine a machine that sorts peaches from large baskets that contain peaches, apples, oranges, and nectarines. The machine determines the size and color of a piece of fruit and then "feels" its surface texture—is it smooth, "fuzzy," dimpled, or something in-between?

Table 1. Fruit-sorting machine with 95 percent sensitivity and 95 percent specificity: 200 pieces of fruit

	Peaches	Apples, Oranges, Nectarines	Total
Fruit tests + as a peach	95 true-positive	5 false-positive	100
Fruit tests − as a peach	5 false-negative	95 true-negative	100
Total	100	100	

For every one hundred pieces of fruit fed into the machine, it will identify peaches with 95 percent accuracy. That is to say, for every one hundred peaches, the machine will correctly identify ninety-five of them. But because the machine is not perfect, and because not every peach has precisely the same texture, color, or size, the machine will misidentify (as apples or oranges or nectarines) the other five. The machine's sensitivity is 95 percent (Table 1).

Specificity is the opposite. If a combination of one hundred apples, oranges, and nectarines were fed into the machine, ninety-five of them would test negative for being a peach, but five would be incorrectly identified as being a peach. The machine's specificity is 95 percent.

A machine that is both 95 percent sensitive and 95 percent specific in sorting peaches might not work well enough for the fruit industry, but such a test would be very accurate in medicine. Let us see what happens with our peach-sorting machine when it is used to test different lots of fruits. The first batch of 1,000 pieces of fruit contains 900 peaches, and the rest is a random assortment of apples, oranges, and nectarines (Table 2). Our machine will correctly identify 855 (95 percent of the 900 peaches), but will misidentify 45 (5 percent of the peaches as apples, oranges, or nectarines). Furthermore, it will correctly identify 95 of the 100 nonpeaches (95 percent of 100 apples, oranges, and nectarines), but it will misidentify 5 of the other fruits as peaches (5 percent of 100).

Of the entire batch of 1,000 pieces of fruit, 860 will have tested positive for being a peach. Of these pieces of fruit that tested positive

Table 2. Fruit-sorting machine with 95 percent sensitivity and 95 percent specificity: Batch 1—1,000 pieces of fruit with 900 peaches

	Peaches	Apples, Oranges, Nectarines	Total
Fruit tests + as a peach	855 true-positive	5 false-positive	860
Fruit tests − as a peach	45 false-negative	95 true-negative	140
Total	900	100	

for a peach, 855 are truly peaches but 5 are apples, oranges, or nectarines. The overwhelming majority (99 percent, or 855 of the 860) of those pieces of fruit that test positive as peaches are peaches—that is to say, the test works very well at identifying peaches in this batch of mostly peaches. The 5 other pieces of fruit that tested positive had false-positive tests. On the other hand, of the 140 pieces of fruit that tested negative for being a peach, 45 of them (32 percent) were in reality, peaches. These 45 peaches had false-negative tests. A negative result in this batch was not very good at truly identifying the non-peaches.

The next batch of 1,000 pieces of fruit to be tested contains only 100 peaches and 900 pieces of apples, oranges, and nectarines (Table 3). Of the 100 peaches, the machine will correctly identify 95 of them (95 percent as peaches) but misidentify 5 of them as nonpeaches. Of the 900 apples, oranges, and nectarines, the machine will correctly

Table 3. Fruit-sorting machine with 95 percent sensitivity and 95 percent specificity: Batch 2—1,000 pieces of fruit with 100 peaches

	Peaches	Apples, Oranges, Nectarines	Total
Fruit tests + as a peach	95 true-positive	45 false-positive	140
Fruit tests − as a peach	5 false-negative	855 true-negative	860
Total	100	900	

identify 855 of them (95 percent) but misidentify 45 of the non-peaches as peaches. For this second batch, there were 140 positive tests, of which 95 (68 percent) were truly peaches and 45 of them (32 percent) were false-positives. In this batch of fruit, a positive test was not nearly as significant; in fact, there was one chance in three that the positive test was a false-positive—that is, that a piece of fruit which tested positive for being a peach was in fact an apple, orange, or nectarine. A negative test in this second batch was strong evidence that the piece of fruit was not a peach; 99 percent of those pieces of fruit that tested negative were truly not peaches.

Why did the machine perform so differently in these two batches of fruit? It is the same machine and still has the same sensitivity and specificity (95 percent) in both cases. The statistical reality is that the same test results will have different meanings depending on the population being tested. Although an individual piece of fruit either is or is not a peach, a test, even a very accurate test, will not be able to make that distinction in every case.

One could imagine that the owner of a fruit company using this machine would not be completely happy with its performance. So the owner directs the engineer to recalibrate the machine so that it correctly identifies a greater percentage of the peaches. The engineer changes the parameters of the machine's texture sensor so that a piece of fruit can be a little less fuzzy and still be characterized as a peach. In this way, she has increased the sensitivity of the machine so that it is more likely that a peach will be classified as such. But what will this do to the specificity?

Now, a peach that had been on the margin—a little smoother than your average peach but a bit rougher than the average apple or nectarine—one that might have been identified by the machine as a nonpeach, will be counted as a peach—that is, more of the non-peaches will test as peaches. So there is a trade-off. The engineer has improved the machine's sensitivity but at the cost of reduced specificity. Now the machine's performance characteristics are a sensitivity of 98 percent and a specificity of 90 percent. More peaches will correctly test positive as peaches but at the same time, more apples, oranges, and nectarines will be misclassified as peaches. On the first

Table 4. Fruit-sorting machine with 98 percent sensitivity and 90 percent specificity: Batch 1—1,000 pieces of fruit with 900 peaches

	Peaches	Apples, Oranges, Nectarines	Total
Fruit tests + as a peach	882 true-positive	10 false-positive	892
Fruit tests − as a peach	18 false-negative	90 true-negative	108
Total	900	100	

batch (Table 4), the machine is even better at finding peaches (882 true-positives as opposed to 855 true-positives). A few more of the nonpeaches will test positive as a peach, but this won't have a big effect because this batch is mostly peaches in the first place. But in the second batch (Table 5), look at those pieces of fruit that tested positive for being a peach. Now, almost half of those positive tests (90 of 188) would be false-positives—apples, oranges, or nectarines that tested as peaches. So trading sensitivity for specificity may help, but it depends on which batch of fruit is being tested.

This basic principle of statistics is true whether applied to peaches, Lyme disease, or heart disease, such as angina pectoris, or simply angina. Angina is usually perceived as a squeezing chest pain or pressure, which typically begins with exertion and is relieved by rest. It is caused by stenosis, or blockage of one or more coronary arteries. Angina is classically what doctors call a "history" diagnosis,

Table 5. Fruit-sorting machine with 98 percent sensitivity and 90 percent specificity: Batch 2—1,000 pieces of fruit with 100 peaches

	Peaches	Apples, Oranges, Nectarines	Total
Fruit tests + as a peach	98 true-positive	90 false-positive	188
Fruit tests − as a peach	2 false-negative	810 true-negative	812
Total	100	900	

which means that one can diagnose it by the history alone. For a patient with epidemiological risk factors and a classical story, the doctor probably doesn't need any other tests. For example, a sixty-year-old man with elevated cholesterol levels, high blood pressure, and diabetes who has central chest tightness that happens only on exertion and is relieved by resting for three or four minutes almost certainly has angina. This is the angina equivalent of an arrow sticking out of the chest.

On the other hand, consider a thirty-five-year-old woman without any of those cardiovascular risk factors who has right-sided sharp chest pain that occurs only intermittently, especially after eating a large meal, but never with exertion. She probably does not have angina.

Suppose that the doctor does a cardiac stress test on these two patients. In this test, the patient walks briskly on a treadmill while having his or her heart function monitored with an electrocardiograph. If there is blockage in a coronary artery, the patient may experience angina and the electrocardiogram may show changes called ST segment depressions. The presence of these symptoms with ST segment depressions would be a positive (abnormal) test. If the sixty-year-old man with a classic history and several risk factors tests negative, there is a good chance that this is a false-negative test. That is to say, the patient truly has angina, but the test does not detect it. If the test is both 95 percent sensitive and specific, and this patient's test is negative, then there is still a 32 percent chance of the test being falsely negative. So this patient with a negative test still has a one in three chance of having angina. This is the same as a peach testing as a nonpeach in the machine testing batch 1 with mostly peaches.

With the thirty-five-year-old woman, if the test is positive—symptoms plus ST segment depressions—there is a 32 percent chance that it is a false-positive test. The woman might not have angina, but the stress test is falsely abnormal. This is akin to the machine testing peaches on batch 2, which contains mostly apples, oranges, and nectarines.

In each of these situations, the doctor would likely do another test that is more sensitive to clarify the ambiguity. Our peach-testing machine and the stress test are both *indirect tests,* that is, the machine is not a human looking at the pieces of fruit, and the stress test does not directly look at the coronary arteries. With peaches, one could always look at the piece of fruit and determine with certainty whether it is or is not a peach. With coronary artery disease, the doctor could do a procedure called cardiac catheterization to directly see whether there is or is not a blocked artery. That is to say, one can adjudicate; there is a so-called gold standard test—a court of final appeal. Because a stress test is neither 100 percent sensitive nor 100 percent specific, there are times when physicians must do the catheterization, which carries more risk, requires more resources, and costs more money.

How does all of this relate to the diagnosis of Lyme disease? As discussed in Chapter 2, physicians diagnose a patient's condition using a variety of methods. Sometimes, all that is required is for the doctor to take a history from the patient. Over the telephone for example, an experienced physician may be able to diagnose a young woman's urinary tract infection or a toddler's middle ear infection with considerable accuracy. In ambiguous cases, the physician will also want to perform a physical examination. On the basis of the history and physical examination, many diagnoses can be reached with a high degree of certainty. Other times, doctors order tests to try to prove (or disprove) a given diagnosis. This can take the form of laboratory tests (analysis of blood or urine), X rays (including CT scan or magnetic resonance imaging), electrical tests (such as electrocardiography for the heart or electroencephalography to measure brain waves), and others.

In the case of infections, the classic means by which doctors diagnose a specific infection is doing a culture—finding the actual bug in the body. Take the example of someone with a sore throat. To see whether the patient has strep throat, the doctor can obtain a throat culture and try to grow streptococcus bacteria. In a classic throat culture, a cotton-tipped swab is touched against the back of the throat and then dabbed onto culture medium that is rich in nutrients that strep bacteria require to grow. If the patient has strep throat, the bacteria will grow, and the culture is reported as positive. But if a virus is causing the infection, the culture will be negative.

Not all tests are so simple or so direct. That same patient with the sore throat may have infectious mononucleosis. To establish this diagnosis, the doctor will send a blood sample to the lab. This test, however, does not measure the actual virus that causes mono, but rather the antibodies that form in the bloodstream as the body fights the infection. Sometimes, the antibodies are not present in measurable quantities during the first week or so of the infection. Therefore, if the test is obtained too soon after the patient becomes ill, it may not be positive yet. This would be an example of a false-negative test—a situation in which the patient truly has the disease but the test result is falsely negative.

Other times, similar blood tests can be positive, but the patient does not have the disease, for example, in the case of the serologic (blood antibody) test for syphilis called a rapid plasma reagin (RPR) test. Patients with all sorts of diseases, primarily involving the immune system, can have false-positive RPR tests—that is, the patient really does not have syphilis but the test result is positive (falsely so).

With regard to Lyme disease, the diagnosis can also be as simple as a history and physical examination. The patient we likened to the arrow in the chest is an example—classic rash in July after a known tick bite in a highly endemic area. Lyme disease is so likely in such a patient that a negative test would still not reduce the likelihood very much. It would therefore be advisable to simply treat such a patient with antibiotics and not bother with a blood test. A false-negative test is more likely than a true-negative test, so why do it at all? Not only is the test only 95 percent sensitive, but there is the additional issue of timing, as mentioned for mono. The blood test for Lyme disease can be falsely negative early on because it can take several weeks for the antibodies to appear in the body in measurable quantities.

The same would be true for a group of patients who had vague symptoms such as aches, pains, and headache but no history of rash or tick exposure, or patients who live in Colorado where Lyme disease is extremely rare, if not absent. In this group of patients, most of whom will not have Lyme disease, a positive Lyme antibody test is far more likely to be falsely positive.

There are different kinds of blood tests for Lyme disease. When Burgdorfer and his colleagues at the Rocky Mountain Laboratories discovered the bacterium, they developed the previously discussed IFA test, which tests for antibodies. Because human interpretation of the test results is involved, this test is not perfectly objective. Furthermore, because the test is not automated, it is very labor intensive. For both of these reasons, researchers developed new tests. These are called the enzyme-linked immunosorbent assay (ELISA) and the Western blot.

19 • Ambiguity in the Lab

We live in a time of instant coffee, fast foods, E-mail communication, and Internet shopping. We have become accustomed to quick results and become impatient waiting for a computer's reply that might take a few more milliseconds than we had anticipated. We expect results to be produced faster and faster. But we demand more than just speed; we also demand accuracy. Furthermore, in medicine, both doctors and patients want another thing: certainty. Unfortunately, given the current status of our science, the lab is simply unable to meet all of these criteria. Although test results are frequently reported as being "positive" or "negative," the work behind that result is not at all so binary.

When a lab performs a test for Lyme disease, the ELISA or the Western blot (or immunoblot) is most likely to be done. Both of these tests measure antibodies in the blood. They are neither actual cultures for *B. burgdorferi,* nor are they assays for the DNA of the spirochete. Antibody tests are indirect tests.

Antibodies, or immunoglobulins, are proteins that the immune system of vertebrates creates to fend off invaders. In the classic science fiction film *Fantastic Journey,* a group of scientists miniaturize themselves and are injected into a dying patient's body to try to save his life. At one point, a character nearly dies after being attacked by anti-bodies. That is the antibody's job—to bind to foreign invaders to slow them down so that other parts of the body's immune system can kill them. When the body's immune system senses foreign sub-stances—such as viruses, bacteria, fungi, or, in the movie, tiny human beings—certain types of white blood cells called lymphocytes begin to produce antibodies. These microorganism-fighting molecules are individually manufactured, such that the body will have one antibody that fights streptococcus, another that attacks the pneumonia bacte-rium, and still another that battles an influenza virus.

It is important to recognize that a "Lyme test"—that is, usually an ELISA or Western blot—will not produce a binary black-or-white result. As discussed in the last chapter, a positive result does not mean conclusively that a person has Lyme disease; nor does a negative result definitely show that a person does not have Lyme disease. If such a test were available, this book might have been satisfactorily concluded two chapters ago.

Many of the ELISAs used to test for Lyme are about 95 percent sensitive and 95 percent specific. This test detects antibodies directed against (that is, antibodies that the body has created to fight) *B. burg-dorferi* in the blood. After the patient's blood is drawn into a glass tube, the red blood cells and other solid elements are allowed to clot, and the serum, or liquid phase, separates. A lab technician puts the glass tube into a powerful centrifuge. As the tube spins, the solid phase migrates toward the bottom of the tube and leaves the amber-colored serum at the top. The serum is the part of the blood that is tested because this is where the antibodies will be, if they are present at all.

The technician places a tiny amount of the serum in small wells, or depressions, on a large plastic plate—something like a muffin tin. Undiluted serum goes in the first well, and then serum diluted with distilled water goes in the following wells—each dilution including more and more water, such that the serial dilutions result in ratios of 1:4, 1:8, 1:16, 1:32, and so forth, of serum to water.

Recall that an antibody binds to an antigen, which is part of the outer surface of the microorganism that the antibody is directed against. They bind together the same way a cordless phone nests in its base; that is, the respective shapes of the phone and the base are manufactured to make a perfect fit so that a telephone made by one company might not fit a base made by a second company. Each antibody binds to a specific antigen. Any given microorganism may possess many different antigens, and the human immune system may generate different antibodies to each of these antigens.

Imagine a microorganism with the shape of an automobile and the parts of the car as antigens. The immune system might develop one antibody against the wheel, another against the taillight, and still another against the side view mirror. The precise shape of the wheel of a Chevy, a Ford, and a Chrysler might all be a little different, each with a specific antibody. At the same time, they might be sufficiently similar so that the antibody to a Ford wheel might react, or bind, to a Chrysler wheel. Furthermore, the wheel of one kind of Ford might be different from another Ford model, but sufficiently similar so that an antibody could mistake the two.

So if one were testing for antibodies to a Ford Explorer, but the patient was infected by a Ford Taurus, the test might be falsely positive. Similarly, if one were testing to see whether a patient was infected by a Ford but the patient was infected by a Chrysler, it is also possible that the test would be falsely positive. This is called *cross-reactivity* and is fairly common in medical diagnostic tests for various infectious agents because to various degrees, their outer surfaces share similar structure, shape, and texture.

Here is how the ELISA works with *B. burgdorferi*. Fixed to the bottom of the wells of the ELISA plate is some *B. burgdorferi*. This is the antigen. The patient's serum sample (or a dilution of the sample) is added to each well. After a short period of time to allow the antibody to bind to the antigen, the wells are washed with distilled water. If there is specific antibody in the specimen being tested that reacts to *B. burgdorferi* attached to the spirochetal antigen fixed to the bottom of the well, the antibody binds to the antigen and remains in the well after washing. If there is none, all the serum is washed away.

The second step of the test involves placing another antibody in the well—this time, an antibody to an antibody, for example, goat antibodies directed against human antibodies. Attached to the goat antibody is an enzyme that has a color that can be measured by a machine—the more antibodies, the more color. Thus, the amount of antibody can be quantified. Unlike the IFA test, the ELISA can be automated; a machine, not the human eye, measures the intensity of color.

The ELISA rapidly replaced the IFA test; however, any hope that this test would be a panacea quickly evaporated. In the mid-1980s, clinicians were beginning to have their doubts about the accuracy of Lyme disease blood assays, and some of them decided to test the hypothesis that different laboratories might be reporting different results. They devised an experiment as clever as it was simple. They took specimens of serum from their patients and split the samples into two portions. Unbeknownst to the laboratories, they sent one portion to one lab and the other portion to a different lab. The results came back different, meaning that the same specimen could test positive in one lab and negative in another. Then the doctors went a step further; they also split specimens and sent both of these identical serum samples to the same lab, labeling the split sample as if each sample were from a different patient. Even more surprising, they found that some specimens would test positive and some test negative at the same lab—and on exactly the same specimen of blood!

These results were published in *JAMA* in 1992, and clearly, Lyme disease testing had developed a black eye. Even though, as a culture, Americans may be able to compromise on speed, and perhaps live with some ambiguity, the notion that these tests were inaccurate was unacceptable.

Other problems with serologic testing go beyond laboratory accuracy. Let us reexamine the issue of cross-reactivity. Recall the analogy of the wheels. It is easy to see that the wheel of a Ford Taurus and a Ford Explorer could be thought to be the same, or very similar. Similarly, a mid-sized Chrysler wheel might look a lot like a mid-sized Chevrolet wheel. In part, this is because engineers have developed structures that work, and they tend to reuse these structures as much as patent law will allow them.

Nature does the same. As scientists increasingly uncover the genetic structure of microorganisms, they are learning that many systems are shared across a large spectrum of the biological universe. For example, if, several hundred thousand years ago, nature found a membrane protein that would allow potassium to be pumped into a cell in a simple bacterium, the gene that coded for that membrane protein would be used in succeeding organisms. A better protein might be found, but that could take thousands of years. Therefore, many microorganisms share similar membrane structures and thus antigenic material. This means that if you get pneumonia from one kind of bacterium, some of the antibodies you develop might cross-react with antigens from other bacteria because they are sufficiently similar, if not identical, to antigens on those other bacteria. There is no problem with the lab here; it is the way nature works. Biologists spent countless hours trying to sort out which of the many surface membrane proteins on *B. burgdorferi* were unique to it. Only then could they develop tests that would be more reliable. If certain proteins (antigens) are found only on *B. burgdorferi* and no place else, then an antibody reaction against that antigen would be very meaningful in diagnosing Lyme disease compared with finding antibodies to an antigen shared widely across bacterial species.

Another problem with antibody testing is perhaps intrinsic to using a test that looks for antibodies rather than for the infectious microorganism itself. As previously discussed, this is the issue of timing. Time is required between the body first becoming infected and the production of antibodies in quantities sufficient to be measured in the laboratory. In the case of Lyme disease, it can take days or weeks for a patient's immune system to begin manufacturing antibodies directed against the invading spirochete. Suppose that a man is bitten by a tick on the Fourth of July. The tick is infected with *B. burgdorferi,* and the man becomes infected and develops EM. He first notices the rash behind his left knee on July 14 and makes an appointment with his doctor, whom he sees on July 16. If the doctor were to draw blood for a Lyme disease blood test at this point (which would be an ELISA looking for antibodies), chances are the test would be negative, or normal. Does this mean the man does not have Lyme disease? Of course not; he does. It simply means that insufficient time has elapsed to allow enough antibodies to form for the test to measure them. This is an example of a false-negative test.

Many of these problems that have existed over the past two decades have been solved by painstaking work done in dozens of research labs by hundreds of scientists around the world. Some of the problems are legacies of biology and statistics that cannot be avoided. The important thing is that both doctors and patients understand what they can know and what they cannot know. It is like navigation at sea. Celestial navigation has one set of limitations—for instance, how the weather affects the navigator's ability to see the stars. The compass and effective methods of measuring time revolutionized the process, but compasses introduce a different set of errors, and clocks are not always true. Successive generations of radar and loran and now global positioning devices allow for even more refined navigation, but all methods have their limitations. If the navigator enters the wrong waypoint or a computer malfunctions, he or she will quickly learn the limitations of these new machines.

Given the problems with the ELISA, the CDC recommended that Lyme testing be done in two steps: a screening ELISA followed, if necessary, by a confirmatory Western blot. All patients with ELISA results that were either positive or equivocal would have their blood tested again by Western blot. If this follow-up Western blot were negative, the test was considered to be negative. If the ELISA were negative, no further testing was recommended and the test results were considered to be negative for Lyme disease.

Like the ELISA, the Western blot tests for antibodies, but it allows the laboratory to find precisely which antigens a patient's blood contains antibodies to—not just whether there are any kinds of antiborrelial antibodies. First, the *B. burgdorferi* is put into a detergent to break up all its proteins. Each of these proteins has different sizes and each has a slight electrical charge. These proteins (antigens) are placed on a gel to which an electrical current is applied. The proteins then migrate across the gel, which is full of nooks and crannies, rather like an English muffin. Because the proteins have different sizes, they move through the gel at different rates, the larger ones moving more slowly than the smaller ones. After a certain amount of time migrating with the electrical current across the gel, the proteins from the *B. burgdorferi* have traveled different distances.

Imagine a massive jungle gym with evenly spaced bars going every which way. A group of people who are four to seven feet tall are instructed to start at one end of the jungle gym and travel through the latticework as far as they can in five minutes toward the other side. In this group of people, ten are exactly four feet tall; ten are exactly four feet, six inches tall; ten are five feet tall, and so on—such that there are seven groups of ten people who are all the same height.

Since the spaces between the bars of the jungle gym are uniform, the smaller people will be able to travel faster across this jungle than the larger, heavier people. When the five minutes are up, the larger people will be closer to the start and the smaller closer to the finish. Assuming that the participants are equal in their abilities, at the end of the five minutes, the seven groups will settle out in seven distinct regions of the jungle gym. If one were to take a picture of the apparatus at the end of the five minutes, it would show seven bands—clusters of people of the same height—interspersed with bare areas of the jungle gym devoid of anyone.

This is what happens to the proteins from the borrelia in the Western blot. They migrate across the gel, through the network of obstructions, at different rates on the basis of their molecular weights. After a specified period of time, the proteins are clustered on the gel at specific regions. They are then transferred (blotted) onto a special kind of white membrane. Specific antibodies (attached to a dye so that they can be seen) will bind to specific borrelial proteins, and colored bands will appear on the white membrane.

Now the laboratory can determine whether the specific antibody in the patient's serum is to a common, cross-reacting antigen or to one that is specific to *B. burgdorferi*. Technicians can measure precisely how many antibodies there are to specific borrelial proteins. Western blots are more time-consuming and expensive than ELISAs and also require some degree of interpretation by a trained individual.

As precise as the Western blot sounds, it still has problems and the results can be controversial. For instance, what strain of *B. burgdorferi* should be used as the antigen? How should it be measured—

by human eye or by a machine using objective criteria? How many bands and which ones should be used to define a sample as positive or negative? Also, just as with the ELISA, timing is still an important issue because time is required for the body to mount a measurable antibody response. Therefore, in 1994 the CDC and governmental agencies held the Second National Conference on Serologic Diagnosis of Lyme Disease in Dearborn, Michigan. Their goal was to better standardize Lyme testing and to improve its accuracy. The CDC held other meetings, called working groups, before the one in Dearborn to give direction to the Dearborn conference, specifically with respect to standardizing the Western blot test. Dearborn was a large meeting and was meant to confer a consensus to the process. The conclusions at the end of this consensus conference, however, had largely been determined before the conference began. This is not uncommon because it is difficult to gather all the players together. And even when that is accomplished, establishing consensus is challenging.

The Dearborn criteria, as they are called, regarding the Western blot define the bands (or antibodies) that one needs to have to call a Western blot positive or negative. These criteria say that for the IgG Western blot, at least five of ten specific bands must be present on the blot. Like any consensus, however, there are dissenting opinions. Two candidate bands on the Western blot—those for outer surface protein (Osp) A and Osp B—were tossed out of the ten by the consensus. Some laboratories and the scientists who run them, however, believe that the Dearborn criteria are too conservative and continue to confer diagnostic importance to bands for Osp A and Osp B. Many dozens of antibodies form against the Lyme spirochete. Why use only the ten that the Dearborn criteria say are significant?

One participant at the Dearborn conference was Dr. Paul Fawcett, head of the Immunology Laboratory at the Alfred Dupont Hospital for Children in Delaware and a specialist in Lyme serologic testing. He has some problems with the Dearborn criteria and also the ability of various laboratories to duplicate them. "The Dearborn criteria was a nice effort," he says, "however, it [the reproducibility of the interpretation] is beyond the technical ability of the manufactured test kits. Some of these bands lie within a millimeter [of each other].

You can't be sure that a band you're calling positive is really the correct one. Look at the CAP [College of American Pathologists] surveys . . . different labs using the same samples and the same strips are getting different results, showing different bands. The manufactured kits contain a [calibrating] test strip that's used [to determine which bands are which]. You can line up the test strip and the strip from the patient, and you have to slide them back and forth to properly line them up."

The Dearborn criteria have other problems. They were worked out in research labs with special expertise; can the test be generalized to other labs? The survey by the College of American Pathologists would suggest not. How intense does the band need to be to be called positive? The Dearborn criteria do not specify this. What about infections with borrelial species that are different from the strain used in the particular test kit being used? This could also be a problem.

The Dearborn conference was a worthy exercise, and the criteria certainly should not be tossed out. Nevertheless, doctors, and patients, must realize that very few tests in medicine are perfect; the wise physician understands the limitations of the diagnostic tests he or she uses—and explains those limitations carefully to the patient. The tests will undoubtedly improve; progress continues to be made. But with these new tests will come new limitations.

20 • A Tick with Two Toxins

The limitations of the diagnostic tests for Lyme disease were just one of several problems that clinicians began to notice. Another phenomenon that physicians treating patients with Lyme disease became aware of was the variability of symptoms. Some patients had worse symptoms than the usual patient with Lyme disease—higher fevers or abnormalities in some of the blood cells, such as severe anemia or low white blood cell or platelet counts. Others had elevated levels of certain enzymes typically released by an inflamed liver that were not classically thought to be a part of Lyme disease. Was this just variability in how Lyme disease can manifest itself? Was it some new disease entirely? Or was it an odd combination of diseases?

In general, doctors look for one disease that best fits a patient's symptoms when making a diagnosis. This is often referred to as applying Ockham's razor. William of Ockham, who lived in the fourteenth century, is credited with saying "Pluralitas non est ponenda sine neccesitate," which translates "Plurality should not be assumed without necessity." With reference to scientific theory, this means that if a given situation has several explanations, all things being equal, the simpler of them is probably the correct one. In the case of medicine, if one disease will adequately explain a patient's array of symptoms, that patient probably has that one disease. For example, a patient who suddenly develops fever, swollen joints, and a skin rash most likely has one disease that underlies all three symptoms, as opposed to three unrelated new diagnoses of a viral infection, osteoarthritis, and eczema.

Of course, the principle of Ockham's razor does not always work, and sometimes patients with multiple symptoms do have multiple diseases. As it turns out, some of the patients who were thought to have bizarre manifestations of Lyme disease were found to have babesiosis or, in Europe, tick-borne encephalitis. These patients did in fact have Lyme disease, but some presented in atypical fashions because some of their symptoms were from Lyme but others were from these other infections.

In Wisconsin and Minnesota, researchers examined the serum of patients with Lyme disease and found that of the ninety-six patients examined, 2 percent were also infected with *B. microti*, the agent of babesiosis in North America. But as these and other scientists began to dig deeper, the story got progressively more complicated. An additional player was introduced on the stage of tick-borne diseases. As with babesiosis, which is more common in animals, this organism's introductory role began as a veterinary illness. A disease of cows called bovine anaplasmosis was described in 1910, followed by heartwater or cowdriosis in 1925. Ten years later, canine ehrlichiosis was described. These were diseases of animals caused by a group of organisms that would become known collectively as *Ehrlichiae*. Ehrlichiae, like the rickettsiae, are obligate intracellular organisms, which means that they must live inside of another cell. In fact, all of them fall under the family Rickettsiaceae in the Linnaean classification system.

The first human ehrlichial disease, Sennetsu fever, was described in the 1950s in Japan, but this disease is very rare and geographically limited. When Lyme disease first reached notoriety, it would be an exceptional nonveterinary doctor who had ever even heard of ehrlichiosis. Even now, it is not especially well-known. In fact, the first human ehrlichial disease—human monocytic ehrlichiosis (HME)—was reported in North America as recently as 1987. Seven years later, in 1994, human granulocytic ehrlichiosis (HGE) was described. The terms *granulocytic* and *monocytic* derive from the fact that the organisms have a tendency to attack certain kinds of white blood cells called granulocytes and monocytes. The story of the ehrlichiae, as well as their nomenclature, is still unfolding and will probably evolve over the course of the next decade, similar to the shifts in the story and nomenclature of Lyme disease.

Patients with HME and HGE have a variety of nonspecific symptoms; they usually have a high fever and chills, often accompanied by headache and severe aching in the muscles. Needless to say, those symptoms could describe dozens of viral illnesses and other diseases as well, making ehrlichiosis difficult to diagnose. Some people with ehrlichiosis have a rash similar to that found with RMSF, but most do not. In fact, ehrlichiosis has sometimes been called "RMSF without the spots." There were certain clues to the diagnosis, such as elevated levels of various enzymes released from liver cells and low blood cell counts.

Gradually, it became clear that some patients could become infected with both *B. burgdorferi* and another tick-borne agent and have some symptoms of one disease and different symptoms of the other. When doctors in Wisconsin and Minnesota examined the serum samples from the ninety-six patients with Lyme disease, they found that 5 percent of them were also infected with the agent of HGE. In two of the patients, they found antibody evidence of infection with all three organisms—Lyme, HGE, and babesiosis! When doctors started by looking at the patients infected with HGE, they found that 15 percent of them had evidence of coinfection with Lyme disease. In Sonoma County, California, other investigators also found serologic evidence of coinfection—with a new species of babesiosis known simply as WA-1 (it was first described in the state of Washington).

On Block Island, off the coast of Rhode Island, other researchers were investigating the same phenomenon. They knew that the tick vectors for both Lyme disease and babesiosis were the same—*I. scapularis*—and they reasoned that some patients were being coinfected by the same tick bite. These investigators went one step further. They identified patients in this study not only by examining stored serum but also by prospectively identifying cases of island residents who were diagnosed with Lyme disease. They then followed these patients carefully by periodically examining them and performing blood tests—such as PCR and antibody tests. They wanted to see whether the patients who were coinfected with both Lyme and babesiosis were sicker than those who were infected only by *B. burgdorferi.*

They found that of the 1,156 patients whose serum they surveyed, 8.4 percent had serologic evidence of babesiosis. They also determined that of the 240 patients diagnosed with Lyme disease, 11 percent were coinfected with babesiosis. When following these patients, they found that these patients were sicker (had more symptoms) for longer and were more likely to have a positive PCR test for *B. burgdorferi* in their blood.

Other investigators, however, looked at the same problem on Nantucket Island and came to the opposite conclusion—that patients with both infections were no more likely to be sicker. How can two groups of scientists study the same phenomenon and arrive at opposite conclusions? There are several possibilities. For instance, the strain of *B. microti* on Nantucket Island may be different from that on Block Island. It is also possible that the doctors came up with different results purely by chance. But the most likely explanation is that the two groups used different methods. The Block Island doctors identified their patients in real time and examined them as their illnesses were evolving, whereas the Nantucket group examined their patients after they had already been ill for awhile, introducing the possibility of bias. The ideal study would be nearly impossible, or at least prohibitively expensive, to perform. Researchers would find all of the patients in real time, they would be examined regularly by physicians who were unaware of the study hypothesis, and no patients would drop out of the study before its conclusion. The researchers would also need to simultaneously follow a control group of healthy individuals.

However one analyzes the data and accounts for the differences, it is clear that some patients in the United States were being infected by more than one organism from a single tick bite. In fact, when other investigators began looking for multiple organisms in the ticks, they found them easily. In one study of one hundred *I. scapularis* ticks from New Jersey, forty-three were infected with the agent of Lyme disease, five with that of babesiosis, and another seventeen with the agent for HGE. Ten of the one hundred contained two agents. Deer ticks infected with both borreliae and ehrlichiae have even been found in Van Cortlandt Park in New York City.

While dual infections were being found in the United States, what was happening in Europe? Dual infections were being reported there, as well, from Italy to Sweden, mostly with ehrlichiosis. But there were additional problems in Europe. For one, the Europeans also have to contend with another tick-transmitted disease called tick-borne encephalitis. Some European patients were being infected with both borrelia and the virus for tick-borne encephalitis. The other issue that is more uniquely European is the fact that in the Old World there are different species of *B. burgdorferi* than in the New World.

When Willy Burgdorfer first discovered the Lyme disease spirochete, he was working with a specific strain of the organism, the B31 strain. However, many other strains of *B. burgdorferi* were subsequently found. A different strain means that there were slight genetic differences between them. As microbiologists in Europe began examining the *B. burgdorferi* on that continent, they made some interesting observations. Just as the clinicians were finding that there seemed to be distinctions between the European and U.S. manifestations of Lyme disease, so, too, the microbiologists were finding genetic differences in the borreliae.

In fact, the genetic distinctions were sufficient enough that scientists thought they were dealing with more than different strains. Therefore, two additional species of borreliae were born. One was named *B. garinii*, after the French physician Garin who described the nervous system findings in 1922. This subspecies was found much more commonly in patients afflicted by neurological manifestations of Lyme disease. The second was named *B. afzelii*, after the Swedish dermatologist Afzelius, who was the first to describe EM. This subspecies was found much more commonly in European patients who had the skin manifestation of ACA. Today, scientists refer to the overarching species as *B. burgdorferi* sensu lato (meaning in the general sense) to encompass all three of these species. The common North American species is technically referred to as *B. burgdorferi* sensu stricto (meaning in the particular or strict sense). Europeans were finding that individual ticks were sometimes infected by more than one species of *B. burgdorferi* sensu lato.

Coinfection is an important concept for three reasons. First, patients who might seem to be having atypical manifestations of Lyme disease might in reality be having typical symptoms of Lyme disease plus typical symptoms of some other, cotransmitted infection. This could lead to obvious confusion as to what disease a patient has or what the manifestations of Lyme disease are (versus those of the coinfecting agent). Second, at least some of the data suggest that those patients who are coinfected have worse symptoms. In fact, of the rare fatal cases of Lyme disease reported in the medical literature, at least one was coinfected with babesiosis and another with tick-borne encephalitis virus. Third, it is possible that coinfecting organisms affect the diagnostic laboratory tests for Lyme disease. Researchers from Westchester County Medical Center in New York found that in patients with HGE only, the majority had positive serologic tests for Lyme disease, including a positive Western blot.

Monocytic ehrlichiosis was being vectored by the Lone Star tick—*A. americanum*—and was found in the same states where that tick was common (Figure 21). Simultaneously, it became clear that patients were being coinfected with the agent that was causing the Lyme-like disease in places such as Georgia and Missouri.

In areas where *I. scapularis* was the vector for Lyme disease, it was also the vector for HGE, so it was not long before patients were being infected by both of these organisms as well. Recall that most patients with Lyme disease in general have low-grade fever and are not especially ill in the acute stages. Now, however, with the issue of coinfection, it was no longer clear which acutely ill patients with Lyme disease just had a bad case of Lyme disease, or which might be coinfected with the agents causing babesiosis or ehrlichiosis.

Furthermore, one disease might not be treated the same way as another disease. A patient treated appropriately for Lyme disease who

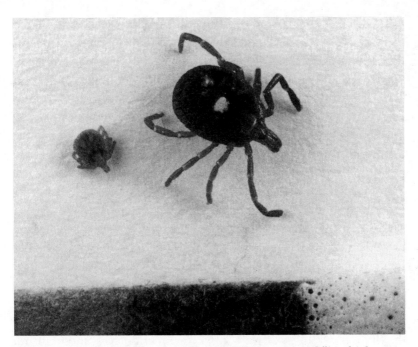

Figure 21. *Amblyomma americanum* tick ("Lone Star tick"), which trans-mits human monocytic ehrlichiosis and a Lyme-like disease (sometimes called Masters' disease) across the southern United States. (Photo by Darlyne Murawski.)

was coinfected with babesiosis would not be receiving appropriate treatment. Someone with coinfecting ehrlichiosis and Lyme disease would be properly treated if they received doxycycline for their Lyme disease but incompletely treated if they got amoxicillin or cefuroxime. This led to new questions. Should coinfection affect how treatment failures for Lyme disease are viewed? Should they affect how the mani-festations of Lyme disease are defined? Imagine a patient who was bitten by a tick that happened to be infected with the agent of HGE and *B. burgdorferi*. The patient has a high fever, a low platelet count, and elevated levels of liver enzymes. Are the blood abnormalities from the Lyme disease or from the ehrlichiosis? Suppose the patient is treated with amoxicillin—a perfectly appropriate antibiotic choice for

Lyme disease—but he or she does not respond to it. Is this a treatment failure of amoxicillin in Lyme disease? If the physician knew that the patient had a coinfection, the answers to these questions would be relatively simple, but if the physician did not know of the coinfection, he or she might draw incorrect conclusions. Unfortunately, as ehrlichiosis is a new disease, physicians often do not think of it, even if they have heard of it in the first place. For those who do know of it, the diagnosis is not easily confirmed, so the average practicing physician must proceed with decisions in the absence of complete data.

Recall that ticks take their blood meal from a vertebrate host in order to transform into the next stage of their life cycle. When they suck the blood of their host, any bacteria, viruses, rickettsiae, toxins, or other such detritus in that host will flow into the gut of the tick indiscriminately. Then, when that same tick goes onto the next stage and bites another vertebrate host, which may be a human being, these freeloading organisms, be they one, two, or more, can then enter the new host. This seems to happen approximately 10 to 15 percent of the time in tick bites, at least in North America. It is important for physicians to recognize this fact so that they can make the best decisions related to diagnosis and therapy.

As previously discussed, the diagnosis of early Lyme disease, at the stage when the patient experiences only EM, is made on the basis of history and physical examination—no lab testing is necessary. If there is a possibility of a coinfecting organism or organisms, however, the physician has to make other decisions. Should she test for babesiosis? Should she test for ehrlichiosis? Should she start empirical therapy for either of those two diseases? Doctors must make these real-life decisions, and they must frequently make them without the luxury of having all of the data they would prefer to have. This story of coinfections is still unfolding, but it is a good example of the effect of emerging diseases on our society and our health, the complexity of our environment, and our interdependence with all living things.

New organisms and diseases are always emerging. While investigators were searching for these organisms in the Midwest, they found a new organism in the genus of bacteria called *Bartonella*. Although this new organism has been found only in mice thus far, it will not be a surprise if it is isolated in humans. We are not, nor probably ever will be, free from infectious diseases.

The past several chapters have illuminated five facts about and issues concerning Lyme disease. First, some manifestations of the disease are still being enumerated, although the more common ones are clearly described. Second, in about one case in eight, coinfection with another tick-transmitted illness may alter or add to those manifestations. Third, diagnostic testing, both for Lyme disease and for these other tick-borne diseases, is imperfect, and doctors need to be knowledgeable about the limitations of diagnostic testing. Fourth, variations of *B. burgdorferi*, or at least very closely related organisms, may be causing a similar disease in geographical areas not traditionally thought to be endemic for Lyme disease. Fifth, the degree to which physicians are knowledgeable about Lyme disease, a malady that was not even in the textbooks when many of them went to medical school, needs improvement. Given these conditions, it is not difficult to imagine that there may be differences of opinion concerning and controversy surrounding what Lyme disease is and what it is not.

21 • Cracks in the Theory

The notoriety of Lyme disease in the United States and the huge amount of research that followed its discovery reenergized the European doctors and scientists. Now they had a firmer base upon which to extend the research that they had been conducting for many decades. The U.S. findings generated new hypotheses that led to new experiments designed to explain the mysteries that remained. For example, why did some manifestations of Lyme disease seem to occur more frequently in Europe and others in the United States? Was it simply that European physicians had not been aware of or looking for them, or were these manifestations truly not occurring as frequently in Europe? Like William of Ockham, doctors prefer simple explanations to more complex ones. It was tempting to believe that Lyme disease in both Europe and the United States were identical illnesses, both caused by *B. burgdorferi*. But instead it was becoming clear that a single unified explanation of events on both sides of the Atlantic was no longer adequate, and as frequently happens in science, the reality turned out to be far more complex than the scientists had initially thought or hoped for.

For instance, there was more genetic heterogeneity in the borrelial species in Europe compared with those in the United States. It was tempting to explain these differences by hypothesizing that Lyme disease was more ancient in Europe and that it had been more recently imported to the New World. This explanation would be consistent with the fact that the disease had been described in Europe long before it was recognized in North America. However, the previously described findings that both ticks and mice from North America and Europe contained DNA from *B. burgdorferi* since the late 1880s made this explanation unlikely.

In fact, scientists did not have an adequate explanation for the differences in the genetic diversity of *B. burgdorferi* on the two sides of the Atlantic. Nor was it certain that the differences in species of the agent accounted for the differences in manifestations of the disease, though it seemed probable. What other differences did these different species of *Borrelia* account for? Would the same antibiotics work? Would the same diagnostic tests apply? If a vaccine for Lyme disease were ever developed, would it be effective on both sides of the Atlantic? These questions now occupied researchers on both continents.

What had originally seemed like a nice, neat, and clean discovery—a tick-borne spirochetal disease that affected the skin, joints, heart, and nervous system—was now becoming mired in a number of complicating realities: problems with serologic testing, the discovery that coinfections by other tick-borne pathogens might cloud the apparent manifestations of Lyme disease, newer symptoms of Lyme disease that were being described even in the absence of coinfections, and increasing evidence in some parts of United States—notably the south central and southeastern states—of newer borrelia that might not even be within the *B. burgdorferi* sensu lato grouping. And now it looked as if the Lyme-causing spirochetes in Europe were different, too!

Ed Masters continued his work in Missouri, and the CDC continued its investigation of the Missouri cases. This epidemiological study was initiated by H. Denny Donnell, the Missouri state epidemiologist; half the patients studied came from Masters's practice. Although Masters and Donnell and the CDC were studying the same phenomenon, they arrived at vastly different conclusions.

The CDC group published its findings in the *Journal of Infectious Diseases* in 1995, concluding that, whatever was happening in Missouri, it was not Lyme disease. The researchers found the incubation period between tick bite and symptoms to be shorter than in patients with Lyme disease. They could not culture *B. burgdorferi* from the skin lesions, as would be expected in a sizable percentage of patients with Lyme disease. They also found negative serologic responses for Lyme disease, using a variety of tests. Although they acknowledged that the Missouri phenomenon could be due to a novel pathogen, they also thought it might be due to a toxin from the tick's saliva or an immunological reaction to the saliva.

When the research was published, Masters and Donnell took the unusual step of declining authorship because they believed that the CDC had approached the investigation with a preconceived conclusion and then made the data fit that conclusion. In a letter to the editor of the journal, Masters and Donnell wrote in 1996 that the CDC's conclusions on the serologic tests were flawed by the criteria they used for interpretation. The tests had been designed for the classic B31 strain of *B. burgdorferi;* those same tests might not perform the same for other strains. The Missouri doctors noted that although the serologic tests were not positive by standard criteria, neither were they negative, and by some published criteria some of the tests would be interpreted as positive.

They also blasted the CDC's methods for determining the incubation period, an important issue since a shorter period favored a toxin-mediated or immunologically mediated mechanism (as opposed to an infectious agent). The CDC used data from questionnaires sent to patients many months after they had been sick, whereas the incubation period recorded in the office charts was recorded contemporaneously and thus was much more likely to be accurate. The CDC data on incubation period was considerably shorter than the data on office charts.

"The most serious and disappointing circumstance was when I caught the CDC red-handed trying to . . . masquerade opinion as data supported by objective and provable facts," says Masters. "The CDC tried to publish that 'qualitative distinctions . . . exist between lesions described in these Missouri patients and EM lesions from pa-tients in known Lyme disease–endemic regions, but based on avail-able photographic evidence, such differences are common (unpub-lished data)' (draft No. 930513). When I read this, as a coauthor, I called the CDC and requested to see the 'unpublished data.' If the CDC could tell these Missouri rashes from Lyme EM just by looking, why were we even bothering to do a study?" That paragraph was dropped from the final paper.

Other reports of an EM-like rash following tick bites began to come from the South. In 1997, similar cases were reported in North Carolina; two years later, the same phenomenon was reported in Georgia and South Carolina. Whatever its cause, something was clearly occurring that either was Lyme disease or looked a lot like it and that was precipitated by a tick bite. The official CDC stance was that Lyme disease was not the cause of this phenomenon, which they refer to as southern tick-associated rash illness (STARI).

Masters points out that the "track record" of the "conventional wisdom" regarding Lyme disease is not very good: "First off, they said it was a new disease, which it wasn't. Then it was thought to be viral, but it isn't. Then it was thought that sero-negativity didn't exist, which it does. They thought it was easily treated by short courses of antibiotics, which sometimes it isn't. Then it was only the *Ixodes dam-mini* tick, which we now know is not even a separate valid tick species. If you look throughout the history, almost every time a major dog-matic statement has been made about what we 'know' about this dis-ease, it was subsequently proven wrong or underwent major modifi-cations."

The implications of whether Lyme disease exists in the South are important. For instance, should cases from these southern states count in official CDC numbers? These official counts can affect the number of research dollars or public education campaigns that are earmarked for Lyme disease. More important, what does a general practitioner do with a patient who walks into the office in July with a rash after a tick bite? Does he prescribe antibiotics or just a steroid cream or antihistamines?

In 1996, Alan Barbour and colleagues reported that they found

DNA evidence of a new borrelia in the Lone Star tick, but they were unable to culture this new bug. They named it *Borrelia lonestarii*. Was this the cause of Lyme disease in the South?

James Oliver at Georgia Southern University agrees that newer observations and experimental data about Lyme disease challenge much of the older dogma. And he believes that the situation in the South is far more complex than in the North. The species of human-biting ticks, the animal reservoirs, and the borreliae themselves are all far more diverse in the South. "Perhaps *B. lonestarii* might cause some cases [of Lyme disease in the South]," he says, "but it is not THE ANSWER to Lyme disease in the South. There is such a gradation of severity of Lyme in patients and such a much greater genetic variability of borrelia in the South that I don't believe there is a simple explanation of one etiological agent."

Humans may seek simple truths, but nature is rarely so accommodating. The more scientists learned, the more complex the world of Lyme disease became. In the mid-1980s, the "party line" had been simple: The bacterial species *B. burgdorferi* was transmitted by the bite of an infected *I. scapularis* tick, and that would lead to infection in some humans. This occurred in endemic areas that were tightly clustered in various parts of the United States and Europe. A blood test could diagnose Lyme disease with a fair degree of accuracy, at least in later stages, and patients who were treated with antibiotics would be rid of the infection.

Into the 1990s, some patients and doctors, however, began having other experiences that led them to question this party line. Polly Murray was one of those people: "There was a widening gulf between what the patients were experiencing and what most of the medical literature was reporting that Lyme disease should be like," she wrote. "Patients were becoming confused and frustrated by the dilemmas in diagnosis. Dr. Steere seemed to be less receptive to what patients were describing, and I felt it more difficult to understand his position on diagnosis, treatment, re-infection, and sero-negative patients." She stated that during a meeting in 1991 in Boston, she and Steere "agreed to disagree over a number of points." In 1987, Steere had moved to Tufts University School of Medicine in Boston. There, he headed his own department and could chart his own course of research and clinical agendas.

Another patient who began to question the current theory was a woman named Karen Forschner, cofounder of the Lyme Disease Foundation. This is how she told her story in public testimony in 1993 in front of the U.S. Senate Committee on Labor and Human Resources: "In 1985, our only child Jamie was born. Unfortunately, I had a bug bite and the full range of Lyme disease symptoms while I was pregnant, and soon after Jamie's birth, his symptoms started. During the pregnancy and after the birth, I was seriously ill with multiple problems including serious joint swelling and pain. Shortly after giving birth, a doctor told me my crippling arthritis was a permanent condition and I would remain on crutches until I required a wheelchair. However, there was this mystery illness called Lyme arthritis, and the doctor offered me two weeks of antibiotics—just in case. If my symptoms went away, I had Lyme. My symptoms temporarily improved but once off treatment, the symptoms came back—in full force."

Eventually, she said, all five of her pets died because of Lyme disease. The heart of her commentary, however, was about her son: "Jamie was the light of our life. . . . By the time he was six weeks old, his health was in question. He had repeated vomiting and eye tremors. By six months old, he was showing signs of brain damage, eye problems, and possible deafness and had ceased to grow properly due to malnutrition. I questioned the doctors about the possibility of whether my son could get Lyme disease from me during pregnancy. I was guaranteed that he could not. Our son was never exposed to ticks and never had a tick bite."

Like Mrs. Murray before her, Mrs. Forschner and her husband, Tom, began doing their own research and concluded that their son had acquired Lyme disease while in the womb. "Then, a doctor saw permanent damage in our son's eyes," Mrs. Forschner said, "damage caused by a congenital spirochetal infection." She and Jamie tested positive for Lyme disease. He was treated with antibiotics on multiple occasions and transiently improved with each course of treatment but would then relapse, sometimes requiring life-support systems.

"But despite the dramatic and documented improvements," Mrs. Forschner's testimony continued, "over the years, local doctors and health officials would repeatedly interfere with our son's re-treatment—as [the doctors believed] Lyme was easily curable. Despite the proven cause and effect of treatment, evaluated by many independent professionals, the label of 'Lyme disease' caused a paranoid behavior to withhold life-saving treatment. When we asked the pediatrician for amoxicillin to give to our son over a three-month period to prevent a relapse, we were told that amoxicillin was dangerous and there was no proof the Lyme bacteria can survive the short-term intravenous medicine he had had while on life support. Two weeks later, we were back to the pediatrician for a potential ear infection. The same pediatrician prescribed the now 'safe' antibiotic amoxicillin to prevent an ear infection that had not yet started. And the prescription was issued in the same dose we had requested for a total of four months."

Mrs. Murray and the Forschners were not the only people to begin questioning the existing theory of Lyme disease. Other patients did as well when they began having symptoms that were not described in the scientific literature. Support groups began to sprout up in areas where Lyme disease was a big problem, such as New York, New Jersey, Connecticut, and Pennsylvania, as well as in Wisconsin and Minnesota. Some individuals began believing that doctors were ignoring evidence that did not fit their point of view.

Some physicians also began to express doubts. One was Dr. Brian Fallon, a psychiatrist at Columbia University's Psychiatric Institute. He knew about Lyme disease because a family member had been affected. Polly Murray had contacted Dr. Fallon in 1991 and told him that she believed many patients with Lyme disease suffered from psychiatric symptoms. She thought there might be a link between the two. On July 29, 1991, Fallon and a second psychiatrist, Dr. Jennifer Nields, drove from Manhattan to Mrs. Murray's house in Connecticut to interview some of these patients. Recalls Fallon: "We interviewed them in her living room, just like we would in a psychiatrist's office, to see what was what. We walked away from that meeting not at all confident that Lyme disease was causing psychiatric symptoms, but it piqued our interest and we designed a survey to test it out."

Their first step was to design and distribute a questionnaire. Through local physicians and Lyme disease support groups, they identified more than 1,100 patients with Lyme disease. The questions on the questionnaire dealt with how the Lyme disease had been diagnosed, results of tests, psychiatric history before the diagnosis of Lyme disease, neuropsychiatric symptoms in the past six months, and other pertinent medical questions. They received 450 responses, not unusual for a survey of this type, especially one that is eleven pages long. Of the 450 patients who responded, 150 had been sero-positive for Lyme. Fallon and Nields focused on these cases because they could be reasonably certain that these sero-positive patients most likely had Lyme disease.

Fallon and Nields knew that any information they gleaned from the patients with Lyme disease would be meaningless without comparing them with control subjects, that is, people who did not have Lyme disease. They also knew that if they compared them with healthy control subjects, some of the responses could be due to nonspecific problems associated with having a chronic disease. They therefore used as their controls people who had other chronic rheumatic diseases, such as lupus and osteoarthritis. "Of those 150 sero-positive patients," Fallon says, "we found that a full 75 percent met criteria for a major depression, most of them for the first time. When we looked at the controls with other chronic rheumatic diseases, only 25 percent did." Following up on these initial findings, Fallon conducted structured interviews with selected patients. He found that some had specific psychiatric diagnoses, such as panic disorder and new-onset mania, which resolved with antibiotic treatment.

These early results got Fallon and Nields started on a line of research that is still going strong ten years later. Fallon became especially interested in neuropsychiatric complications of Lyme disease in children.

Other physicians also noted that some patients had persistent symptoms after so-called standard antibiotic therapy. One of these doctors was Kenneth Leigner, an internist in Armonk, New York. Leigner began to practice in Westchester County in 1985. Trained in internal medicine and critical care, Leigner recalls, "My getting into Lyme disease was pure chance. . . . I saw a few patients, like everybody else here, and became interested in it. What struck me the most was that patients didn't seem to fit the book. They kept relapsing when I tried to stop treating them. I used the standard 14- to 21-day treatment . . . but the patients would stay sick. So I'd extend treatments longer and longer. And a lot of times even then, they'd get sick when I stopped treatment."

Leigner tells of one illustrative case in which his patient had an undiagnosed neurological illness for about two years. She experienced muscle spasticity, slurred speech, and some problems with her cranial nerves. An extensive evaluation did not disclose the cause of his patient's symptoms. Among other abnormalities, she had lymphocytes in her spinal fluid. Tests for Lyme disease were negative. "The bottom line was that we went through this whole differential diagnosis of about twenty things and none of them panned out," Leigner recalls. "We had excluded just about everything else, and Lyme was treatable and she lived in an endemic area and there was no other explanation. We had no real proof of Lyme. With no real conviction that it was Lyme disease, we just treated her empirically with cefotaxime."

The cefotaxime, a powerful antibiotic with activity against *B. burgdorferi*, did not seem to change the cell count in her spinal fluid, but Leigner persisted and used an oral tetracycline derivative for four more months. "To be honest, neither seemed to have a lot of impact," he remembers. A few months later, in December 1991, he repeated a spinal tap to test her spinal fluid. "I was doing some work for the CDC; they were supplying me with culture media, so then I tapped her again and I got a call a few weeks later from the CDC. There were spirochetes growing [in the spinal fluid]. I knew it was *Borrelia burgdorferi*."

Now that Leigner had a definitive diagnosis, he treated for longer periods of time. Finally, for the first time in several years by that point, the cells in her spinal fluid cleared. Leigner points to other similar patients, who, while they did not have positive cultures like the first patient, have had chronic problems from Lyme disease that he believes require longer courses of antibiotics than what are conventionally prescribed.

Gradually, a clear-cut schism arose between one group of doctors and another, along with various patient advocacy groups. In 1993, this schism reached sufficient proportions that the U.S. Senate Health and Human Services committee, chaired by Ted Kennedy, held hearings on the subject.

The biology of the bug is partly to blame for this controversy. *Borrelia burgdorferi* is not the same as the staphylococcus or the pneumonia bacterium, both of which strike rapidly, inflict their damage, and then either vanquish or are defeated by the host. Rather, *B. burgdorferi* can fight something more akin to guerrilla warfare. Doctors have cultured the bacteria from patients' skin more than ten years after their initial infection.

Recall Joe Dowhan, the Connecticut biologist who brought the first *I. scapularis* tick into Steere's clinic at Yale back in 1976. "I was never treated with antibiotics because they didn't have a clue back in 1976 what it was," recalls Dowhan. "All I took was aspirin. Never cortisone. I had migratory joint pain and swollen joints; eventually the rash itself went away. Here I was in the heart of a field season and by the beginning of July [of 1976], I was crawling up the stairs to get home. The other biologists were finally telling me to just stay in the car because it was slowing everyone down. I was incapacitated with the disease. But eventually it petered out." Over the years, he would periodically get blood tests, and when the spirochete was discovered, Steere offered him antibiotics. At the time, now years after his initial infection, Dowhan felt perfectly well, except for occasional joint pain, so he declined taking a long course of antibiotics.

Dowhan's work with the U.S. Fish and Wildlife Service took him to Washington, Nevada, and California, where he would occasionally feel sore joints. In 1989, he returned to Connecticut. "In 1990, I started feeling a generalized malaise, a real fatigue, headaches, neck aches," he says. "I just had overwhelming fatigue, unrelated to exercise. I would find myself at two in the afternoon absolutely needing to drop my head on the desk. I just couldn't move. I'd come home. My pockets would be stuffed with notes [to myself]; I was having a difficult time remembering things and getting dinged by my bosses for not following through with things, not even remembering phone conversations with them. Elise [a research assistant of Steere's] would call from time to time asking how I was feeling. And I said, 'Just these past few months now, I've been feeling really worn out.' And there were no joint symptoms, which is why I made no association with [Lyme disease]."

Because of these new symptoms, Dowhan went in for a checkup and was found to have neurological Lyme disease—thirteen years after his initial infection!

22 • Another Paradigm

In the fourth century B.C., Aristotle proclaimed that the Earth was the immobile center of the universe, with the sun, moon, stars, and other heavenly bodies spinning around it in perfect circular orbits. Two centuries later, the Greek astronomer Claudius Ptolemy tinkered a bit with Aristotle's view of the cosmos, but left its geocentric foundation intact. Ptolemy's system predicted the positions of the stars and planets with a modicum of accuracy, and it adequately explained many of the astronomical observations that had been made at that time, making it superior to competing theories. It was, however, by no means perfect. Over the ensuing centuries, Ptolemy's successors worked on these minor errors in the predicted positions of various heavenly bodies, making small adjustments to Ptolemy's theory— a nip here and a tuck there. Each adjustment would improve one particular prediction but invariably throw off another. Over centuries, Ptolemaic theory, taken with all of these "adjustments," became unmanageably complex.

A geocentric universe seemed to be a self-evident truth. After all, when standing on the ground, one does not feel a sensation of movement. If one throws a ball straight up in the air, it drops directly back down into the thrower's hand. The sun always rises in the east and sets in the west.

This was the prevailing wisdom until the Polish astronomer Nicolaus Copernicus questioned it. Copernicus made careful observations about the movements of Jupiter, Saturn, the sun, and the moon and found that a geocentric universe was not consistent with his observations. Copernicus had some trepidation about announcing his new theory, which not only contradicted prevailing wisdom, but more importantly, the truth according to Holy Scriptures. "For a long time, I reflected on the confusion in the astronomical traditions concerning the derivation of the motion of the spheres in the universe," he wrote. "I began to be annoyed that the philosophers had discovered no sure scheme for the movements of the machinery of the world, created for our sake by the best and most systematic Artist of all. Therefore, I began to consider the mobility of the Earth and even though the idea seemed absurd, nevertheless I knew that others before me had been granted the freedom to imagine any circles [orbits] whatsoever for explaining the heavenly phenomena."

Copernicus published his findings in *De Revolutionibus Orbieum Coelestium* just before his death in 1543. He wrote the book in Latin, the language of scientists, not of the common people. He was not trying to persuade the general public and was acutely aware of the risk he was taking in questioning the Church: "The scorn which I had to fear on account of the newness and absurdity of my opinion almost drove me to abandon a work already undertaken." Dava Sobel chronicles this scientific history in her book *Galileo's Daughter*. She also emphasizes that Galileo, when he was teaching astronomy in 1592, still taught the classic Aristotelian viewpoint, despite his being aware of Copernicus's theory. In 1597, just five years later, he wrote to a friend that the Copernican view of the universe was "much more probable than that other view of Aristotle and Ptolemy." Gradually, over the ensuing decades, Galileo accumulated more and more evidence in the form of direct observations that the geocentric explanation of the ancients was wrong.

Eventually, Galileo openly challenged the prevailing wisdom, and he did so in the context of a Church that was all-powerful and that vigorously clung to the old Aristotelian-Ptolemaic explanation of the universe. Galileo was silenced in 1616, when the Church made it clear to him that Copernican thinking was contrary to Holy Scriptures and therefore heretical. At that point, Galileo stopped broadcasting his views, at least temporarily. Then, in 1632, he published his *Dialogue.* Understanding that the Church might have problems with its contents, Galileo was careful to have members of the Church Inquisition review the material before its publication. That body officially approved the manuscript, but when the five-hundred-page book came out and was clearly sympathetic to the Copernican view, Pope Urban VIII reversed himself. Galileo was arrested and tried in 1633. Essentially, he remained under house arrest until he died in 1642.

Science and scientists exist in the context of the world and a specific culture. This was no different in the sixteenth and seventeenth centuries than it is now. Three hundred years ago, the Catholic Church had enormous influence on European scientific thought; today, perhaps the NIH, pharmaceutical companies, and other organizations that fund research fill that earlier role. In another one hundred years, perhaps it will be something else.

In 1962, Thomas S. Kuhn published a book titled *The Structure of Scientific Revolutions,* which sold more than one million copies. In that book about the history of science and the development of scientific thinking, Kuhn asserts that science advances not as an orderly, cumulative evolution of ideas, one placed neatly atop the other, but by "revolution," by quantum leaps of thought. A new instrument (a microscope or telescope, for example) or a new genius (Copernicus or Galileo) may precipitate these revolutions. Moreover, Kuhn argues that these advances occur within a sociopolitical context. His book popularized the word *paradigm* and the phrase *paradigm shift.* Scientists explain natural phenomena using one theory (or paradigm) and then try to "fit" the data (their observations) into that paradigm.

As to the nature of the cosmos, Kuhn wrote: "By the thirteenth century, Alfonso X could proclaim that if God had consulted him when creating the universe, he would have received good advice. In the sixteenth century, Copernicus' co-worker, Domenico da Novara, held that no system so cumbersome and inaccurate as the Ptolemaic had become could possibly be true of nature. And Copernicus himself wrote in the preface to the *De Revolutionibus* that the astronomical tradition he inherited had finally created only a monster. By the early sixteenth century, an increasing number of Europe's best astronomers were recognizing that the astronomical paradigm was failing in application to its own traditional problems. That recognition was prerequisite to Copernicus' rejection of the Ptolemaic paradigm and his search for a new one."

A physicist, Kuhn uses many examples to illustrate paradigms from that branch of science. Examples of paradigm thinking, however, also exist in the field of medicine. Lord Kelvin, for example, a prominent scientist at the turn of the century, denounced the discovery of X rays by Wilhelm Roentgen "as a hoax." And consider the case of the Hungarian physician Ignaz Semmelweis. In July 1846 he began serving in the Vienna Maternity Hospital, probably the largest maternity hospital in the world at the time. The hospital was divided into two parts—first clinic and second clinic. Admissions were alternately assigned to the two clinics depending on the day of the week. Physicians and medical students staffed the first clinic, and midwives staffed the second clinic.

Semmelweis noticed, as had other doctors before him, that the mortality rate at the physician-run clinic was almost triple that of the midwife-run clinic. The death rate in the former was 98.4 per 1,000 births, and it was only 36.2 per 1,000 at the latter. In one year, 1846, the death rate was fully six times higher in the physician-run clinic. Most of the deaths were from puerperal or childbed fever. Nobody at the hospital had been able to explain this difference, although Eduard Lumpe, who was at the Viennese Maternity Hospital just before Semmelweis, had blamed the problem on atmospheric and "miasmatic" conditions. The fact that the two clinics were adjacent to one another, and therefore shared the same atmosphere, did not seem to affect his assessment.

For women who became ill, physicians prescribed various "antiphlogistic" treatments such as bloodletting, dietary restrictions, purgatives, and skin lotions to cool the body. K. Codell Carter, who translated Semmelweis's 1861 work *The Etiology, Concept, and Prophylaxis of Childbed Fever* into English, quotes one practitioner of the time who, when he observed symptoms of puerperal fever, "immediately ordered 'eight or a dozen leeches to be scattered over the abdomen.'" Bloodletting by leeches was consistent with the medical paradigm of the era, which had not yet been replaced by Louis Pasteur's and Joseph Lister's germ theory.

Semmelweis found an important clue when a friend of his, Professor Jakob Kolletschka, died from a wound that he received while performing an autopsy. On examination, his tissues showed the same pathologic lesions as the women with puerperal fever had. Both were contaminated by "decaying organic matter," the best vocabulary that Semmelweis had in this pre–germ theory era. "I was forced to admit that if [Kolletschka's] disease was identical with the disease that killed so many maternity patients," he wrote, "then it must have originated from the same cause that brought it on in Kolletschka."

Semmelweis concluded that medical students who were examining the women in the first clinic after conducting autopsies were transferring a septic and contagious agent from the autopsy room to the patients. He ordered students to wash their hands in a solution of chlorine, and the mortality rate fell over two years. The conclusion that puerperal fever could have the same root cause whether it occurred after childbirth or after getting nicked by a contaminated scalpel was as radical to mid-nineteenth-century physicians as the idea of a non-geocentric cosmos was to sixteenth-century astronomers or theologians. And Semmelweis paid the same price as Galileo. His theory was largely rejected. He suffered increasing emotional difficulties and died in 1865.

Readers may want to believe that scientific thinking has evolved over the past 150 years such that new ideas are more readily accepted on the basis of their underlying science. But that isn't necessarily the case, as the shifts in thought concerning peptic ulcer disease discussed in Chapter 13 show. The "truth" that acid caused ulcers was as "self-evident" to physicians in the 1970s as a geocentric universe was to seventeenth-century Florentine scientists. That is why it was so difficult for Dr. Barry Marshall to persuade his medical colleagues that a bacterium, not stress and diet, caused ulcers and that these patients could be cured not by antacids but by antibiotics.

There are other contemporary examples of new concepts that defied the conventional wisdom, such as kuru and Jakob-Creutzfeldt disease, which are caused by a novel class of infectious particle called prions, whose properties are still being sorted out by scientists. Another new theory suggests that infection with chlamydia may in part be responsible for causing heart disease. New ideas are constantly being generated and tested in modern science; it is an intrinsic part of the process of scientific growth. At the same time, many of these new ideas are scoffed at when first introduced.

By the early 1990s, enormous advances had been made in the study and understanding of Lyme disease—not only in terms of what physicians knew about the disease but also in terms of understanding Lyme disease as a public health problem. Nevertheless, by the early years of the last decade of the twentieth century, Lyme disease was developing a political twist, with two main "parties," or camps, that had differing points of view, mostly concerning the treatment of Lyme disease.

These two camps are descriptively called *conventional* and *alternative*. Neither term is meant in a pejorative sense; "conventional" simply describes the fact that these people support the treatment standard that most organizations and physicians support. "Alternative" describes the fact that some medical practitioners and community-based patient groups believe that there is another, more effective way to treat some patients with Lyme disease. This does not necessarily refer to "alternative" medicine in the sense of herbal remedies, acupuncture, biofeedback, and the like. It is simply a competing paradigm.

Allen Steere typifies the conventional camp. Of mainstream physicians and scientists, the majority would agree with Steere's view of Lyme disease. The alternative camp is typified by Dr. Joseph J. Burrascano Jr., an internist based in Long Island who specializes in Lyme disease and who has written many treatment guidelines for the disease. The view, or paradigm, of the conventional camp can be summarized thus:

- EM is seen in 90 percent or more of patients with Lyme disease.
- Lyme disease can be diagnosed relatively easily.
- Currently available blood tests are highly accurate in late-presenting cases.
- Existing treatment works in most patients.
- Antibiotic therapy beyond one month (or at most two months in resistant cases) is unnecessary and possibly harmful.

The paradigm of the alternative camp is noticeably different:

- EM occurs in only approximately 50 percent of cases.
- The currently available serologic tests are inaccurate in as many as 35 percent of late-presenting cases.
- Many patients will fail to respond if given medication that follows existing treatment recommendations.
- Long-term antibiotic therapy is frequently necessary to control, if not to cure, Lyme disease.

During the 1980s and 1990s, people with Lyme disease began to come together in support groups all over the country. Lyme disease–related Web sites also sprang up. An Internet search for "Lyme disease" on October 30, 2001, yielded more than 171,000 hits. These sites may be associated with universities or various Lyme disease organizations, or they may be the Web sites of individual patients or support groups. Emotions can run high; the language on some of these sites is quite provocative. And the accuracy of the statements on some of these sites must be questioned. Web-based information in all fields has exploded over the past decade; however, there is no arbiter for accuracy, and considerable variability in quality exists.

In 1990, Leonard Sigal, a Yale-trained rheumatologist philosophically aligned with the conventional camp, published a paper in the *American Journal of Medicine* reporting on the first one hundred patients who came to his Lyme disease clinic at the Robert Wood Johnson Medical School in New Jersey. Sigal concluded that only thirty-seven of those patients actually had Lyme disease. Twenty-five of the one hundred were diagnosed with a malady called fibromyalgia.

Three years later, in 1993, Steere and colleagues published a similar paper of their experience at the New England Medical Center in Boston. Steere reported on nearly eight hundred patients who had been referred for probable Lyme disease. Steere thought that Lyme disease was causing the symptoms in only 23 percent of that group. He, too, diagnosed fibromyalgia, as well as chronic fatigue syndrome, in many of these patients. Steere also claimed that patients who were sero-positive in other labs were sero-negative in his lab.

Both Sigal and Steere believed that most of the courses of antibiotics that had been given to these patients had been administered in error and that the most common reason for lack of improvement after antibiotic treatment was the incorrect diagnosis of Lyme disease in the first place. The alternative camp rallied against these articles, especially Steere's, which was titled "The Overdiagnosis of Lyme Disease" and was published in the high-profile journal *JAMA*.

Just four months later, on August 5, 1993, the U.S. Senate Committee on Labor and Human Resources conducted hearings to examine "the adequacy of current diagnostic measures and research activities in the prevention and treatment of Lyme disease." The hearings had originally been scheduled for the week before but were changed at the last minute, even after many people had traveled to Washington to testify. Because many of them could not return to the capital on August 5, their testimony was included in written form. Counting these written testimonies, more than four hundred statements were placed into evidence.

During governmental hearings, panels of four or five witnesses often make prepared statements and are then questioned by members of Congress. Each panel usually consists of four or five people sitting at a long oak desk behind microphones and identification placards. Perhaps nowhere was the gap between the thinking of the conventional and alternative camps more apparent than when the second panel of witnesses gave its testimony. Both Allen Steere and Joseph Burrascano were seated on that panel.

Burrascano began: "There is in this country a core group of

university-based Lyme disease researchers and physicians whose opinions carry a great deal of weight. Unfortunately, many of them act unscientifically and unethically. They adhere to outdated, self-serving views and attempt to personally discredit those whose opinions differ from their own. They exert strong, ethically questionable influence on medical journals, which enables them to publish and promote articles that are badly flawed. They work with government agencies to bias the agenda of consensus meetings and have worked to exclude from those meetings and scientific seminars those with ultimate [sic] opinions.

"They feel that when the patient fails to respond to their treatment regimen, which is a common occurrence, it is not because the treatment has failed, but because they have developed a new illness, what they call the 'post Lyme syndrome.' They claim that this is not an infectious problem but a rheumatological or arthritic malady due to activation of the immune system.

"Because of this bias by this inner circle, Lyme disease unfortunately is both underdiagnosed and undertreated in this country to the great detriment of many of our citizens."

Then Steere, seated only two seats to Burrascano's left and testifying just a few minutes later, spoke: "There is no evidence that many months or even years of antibiotic therapy are necessary to eradicate the Lyme disease spirochete. Because of the success of early antibiotic therapy in acute Lyme disease, chronic active Lyme disease has become an unusual illness. However, infection with B. burgdorferi may occasionally trigger several puzzling syndromes that appear to continue after apparent eradication of the spirochete. . . . we have reported, as have others, that infection with B. burgdorferi may trigger chronic fatigue syndrome or a chronic pain syndrome called fibromyalgia. In our experience, these patients are not helped by further antibiotic therapy.

"Finally, it is important to point out that chronic Lyme disease has become a catch-all diagnosis for a number of confusing and difficult-to-treat conditions. Of 788 patients evaluated at our center in the last five years who were referred with a presumptive diagnosis of chronic Lyme disease, . . . we thought that the majority had other illnesses, particularly chronic fatigue syndrome or fibromyalgia, not triggered by spirochetal infection."

This counterpoint was not lost on the senators. At one point during the testimony about diagnostic testing, Senator Howard Metzenbaum of Ohio interrupted Burrascano and said, "This gentleman [speaking of Steere] says exactly the opposite of what you said." Burrascano and Steere then debated the relative merits of serologic testing for Lyme disease. At several points during their testimony, the crowd, filled with patients from Lyme disease support groups, alternately cheered or booed.

One of the biggest differences between the conventional and alternative camps regards the duration of antibiotic treatment for all stages of Lyme disease, but especially for late-stage Lyme disease. It became clear in the late 1980s and early 1990s that some patients, especially those who had been diagnosed and treated late in the natural course of infection with B. burgdorferi, developed chronic symptoms. On this point, nearly everyone agreed. At some time after being treated for Lyme disease, these patients experienced pains, numbness, and sleep disturbances. They also had trouble concentrating, as well as a profound sense of fatigue, often requiring twelve to eighteen hours of sleep per day.

There are only so many logical possibilities to explain such persistent symptoms. The alternative camp believed that the correct explanation was persistent infection with B. burgdorferi. To use a war analogy, this would be comparable to the fact that all of the enemy soldiers had not been eliminated. They might have been hiding in buildings or in caves, and when the friendly troops left (when the antibiotics were stopped), the enemy (the spirochetes) reemerged to wage war on the body.

Another explanation is that the symptoms could be the result of permanent tissue damage from the initial infection. Even though the spirochete was gone, the damage left behind could still cause nerve cells to misfire or other injured cells to malfunction. This would be akin to having persistent problems after a battle because some of the infrastructure had been permanently damaged. If the war damaged the train tracks and the electrical and water systems in a region, persistent "symptoms" in the war-ravaged areas would continue for some time until these services were restored, even though the enemy had been vanquished.

A third possibility is that the problem could be an autoimmune response triggered by molecular mimicry. Rheumatic fever is such an example. The streptococcus bacteria may be killed, but antigens on the surface of the bacteria share common shapes with antigens on host cells in the heart and nervous system. Thus, the heart valves and parts of the nervous system can be attacked—not, however, by the bacteria, but by the patient's own lymphocytes and antibodies. This is like collateral, unintended damage in a war. The host defenses target the spirochetes, but because some of the good guys (that is, the cells in the nervous system) have a similar appearance, they are attacked as well. Because these cells persist after the real enemy has been wiped out, they may cause ongoing problems in identification of who is enemy and who is not.

Still another possible explanation for these persistent symptoms is that Lyme disease triggers a second process—such as fibromyalgia, chronic fatigue syndrome, anxiety, or depression. This would be similar to the effect of a war on the economy. The bombs or missiles do not directly affect the economy, but the shifts in consumer and defense spending or consumer confidence do. The war is over, but this new problem, triggered by the war, is set in motion and causes its own set of problems that have their own set of solutions. Similarly, the immune system could be nonspecifically "revved up," and the immune cells or their by-products could damage host cells. This is the likely mechanism for some patients with persistent joint swelling in Lyme disease. The war analogy here is that army or intelligence personnel have been activated, but after the war is over, they persist in their activity, sometimes a bit overexuberantly.

Even another explanation for persistent symptoms after treatment for Lyme disease is that a second disease is present—either a coinfected tick-borne organism or a second disease altogether. To continue the war analogy—there are two factions of the enemy; one has been wiped out, but a second faction (the coinfecting organism) is still fighting. Or in the case of a second disease, there is in fact a new war against a different enemy. Although patients can be reinfected by a second tick bite, these arguments largely apply to patients with persistent symptoms from a single initial infection.

Of course, the possibility also exists that one of the above mechanisms is operating in some patients, with others relevant to other patients, or that multiple mechanisms are at work in any individual patient.

The conventional camp believed that the active infection with *B. burgdorferi* had been eliminated in these patients and that these symptoms were from a variety of causes—most commonly fibromyalgia or chronic fatigue syndrome. The alternative camp believed that these patients still harbored active infection with the Lyme spirochete. It is easy to see why these two groups' ideas on therapy diverged in such opposite directions. If these persistent symptoms were being caused by fibromyalgia or chronic fatigue syndrome, then the treatment should be directed against those problems. But if symptoms were due to persistent infection, then more antibiotics would be a reasonable option.

The conventional researchers could find no evidence of the spirochete (by culture) or its DNA (by PCR) after one to two months of therapy. They believed that any symptoms that persisted, at least in most cases, were not due to the persistence of living borreliae. The alternative camp felt that to say that one's Lyme disease is cured and to pronounce any new symptoms to be due to a new disease—chronic fatigue or fibromyalgia—was making a big assumption, pointing to three lines of evidence against this assumption.

First was their own "in-the-trenches" experience with large numbers of patients whom they were seeing with severe, persistent symptoms that seemed to improve after repeated courses of antibiotics. The second line of evidence was experimental. Experiments suggested that *B. burgdorferi* could be enveloped by lymphocytes and macrophages or become cloaked by the lymphocyte cell wall, thus helping it evade the patient's immune system. Other experiments showed that *B. burgdorferi* could live inside cells even when those cells were bathed in otherwise toxic amounts of the antibiotic ceftriaxone. Still others showed that the spirochetes could change their outer coat membranes, typical of borreliae, and some have suggested that *B. burgdorferi* can morph into a dormant form. The third line of evidence in support of the notion that live *B. burgdorferi* remained in chronically symptomatic patients was the occasional case reports of actual patients, such as Dr. Leigner's, who were treated with "curative" amounts of antibiotics but then later had a positive culture for *B. burgdorferi.*

The conventional camp accused the alternative doctors who were prescribing long courses of intravenous antibiotics of profiteering from these desperate patients, either from the fees they received from the patients themselves or from kickbacks from the companies behind home intravenous therapy. Likewise, the alternative camp accused the conventional doctors of lining their pockets with consulting income from big insurance companies, which favored shorter courses of antibiotics because it would cost them less money. They also believed that the conventional physicians had cornered the market on NIH grant money.

All this controversy led the different groups of physicians to consider different treatments.

23 • Therapeutic Adventures

Periodically, Dr. Burrascano published sets of "diagnostic hints and treatment guidelines" for Lyme disease on his Web site. The eighth edition, which was copyrighted in June 1993, said this about the duration of antibiotic treatment for Lyme disease: "We found conclusively that the duration of treatment is just as important as the choice of antibiotic. If treatment with antibiotics is discontinued before all symptoms of active infection have cleared, a relapse usually occurs, especially in sicker patients. All patients respond differently, and therapy must be individualized. The average duration of successful treatment of advanced cases is four months for males and six months in hormonally active females."

In the appendix to that document, Burrascano explains his rationale. In 1987, he studied twenty-six patients with Lyme disease who had positive cultures for *B. burgdorferi*. They were treated for fourteen days with the antibiotic ceftriaxone. Most of the patients initially responded, but Burrascano found that they later relapsed. If they were treated for longer, however, the success rate of treatment rose.

Long-term antibiotic treatment, however, has its negative aspects. Cost is one. Although it varies by region and by antibiotic, the price for intravenous antibiotics is between $1,000 and $2,500 per week. On the global end of the negative spectrum, as previously mentioned, antibiotic use can lead to the creation of more powerful germs, as they become resistant to antibiotics to which they are exposed frequently and over time.

Then there are specific potential adverse effects on individual patients. Long-term intravenous medications require special intravenous lines to be inserted beneath the patient's skin near the front of the shoulder. The long plastic catheter is snaked through the soft tissues of the chest wall and then passed into a large vein, such as the subclavian vein beneath the collarbone. Immediate risks from needle placement are unusual and generally can be treated easily. Maintaining a long-term catheter, however, can lead to infections in the bloodstream and to clots that form on the catheter. These serious infections occur when bacteria that normally live on the skin breach this important barrier to microbial invasion. Furthermore, having a catheter inside a vein creates an artificial pattern of blood flow, and the material that the catheter is made of can be thrombogenic—that is, it can cause blood to clot.

Besides the risk of the catheter, there is risk from the long-term antibiotics themselves. Patients can develop fungal infections or antibiotic-associated bowel inflammation (colitis) from taking antibiotics. One thirty-year-old woman died from massive fungal infection caused by an intravenous catheter that had been in place for more than two years so that she could receive ceftriaxone for Lyme disease. With the ceftriaxone, there was another problem. Occasional patients receiving long-term intravenous ceftriaxone developed gallstones and inflammation of their gall bladders, sometimes so severe as to require surgical removal of that organ. In one hospital in central New Jersey, CDC investigators found a cluster of these patients with gall bladder problems, many of them children, in whom gallstones and gall bladder surgery are distinctly uncommon. To make matters worse, the CDC investigators believed that many of these patients never had Lyme disease in the first place. The conventional camp argued that these patients should never have received these prolonged courses of antibiotics. Of course, disagreement also existed over the accuracy of the diagnosis of Lyme disease in these patients.

In 1992, Lora Mermin, a Wisconsin woman with Lyme disease, gathered, edited, and published a compilation of articles, stories, and vignettes that she titled *Lyme Disease 1991: Patient/Physician Perspectives from the U.S. and Canada.* One contributor, a man whom she identified as Craig Walker, recounted a telephone call that he and his wife received from their daughter Mary in late June 1990. At the time, Mary was a doctoral student at Yale and she had been ill with something—the diagnosis of Lyme disease was still unconfirmed—for about a year and a half. As Walker told the story: "In a strained voice she said that she was tired of all of this and that she had decided to try the radical treatment suggested by Dr. Henry Heimlich in a letter to the *New England Journal of Medicine* in April 1990. If we would not help her, then she would sell her car and use the funds to go to Mexico to try and get malaria."

Heimlich is a household word because of the bear hug–like maneuver he described to relieve upper airway obstruction in a choking victim. Trained as a thoracic surgeon, he has also developed an operation to replace the diseased esophagus, invented a one-way flutter valve used to treat victims of collapsed lungs, and designed other medical devices, all of which bear his name. In 1982, he established the Heimlich Institute to conduct scientific, cultural, and social research into issues of importance to the medical and scientific community. He became interested in Lyme disease after watching a television program about it. As the show progressed, describing the course of the disease—a skin lesion that could be treated with antibiotics but if left untreated could result in neurological symptoms—he thought, "This is beginning to sound like syphilis."

In 1990, he wrote the letter to the editor that Mary Walker had read. In that letter, he suggested that malariatherapy—intentionally contracting malaria to treat a disease—might be useful to treat chronically symptomatic patients. While the notion of intentionally infecting someone with malaria may seem preposterous, malariatherapy actually had a long and honorable past.

To understand this history, one must understand syphilis in its historical context. Today, syphilis can be considered a sexually transmitted disease curable with a shot of penicillin, but at the turn of the last century, it was a devastating illness whose cause was unknown. The early manifestations—skin lesions, fever, swollen lymph glands, and others—could make one sick enough; however, the later tertiary stages were an enormous public health issue. Late-stage syphilis often involved the cardiovascular system, especially the aorta, and the central nervous system, both the brain and spinal cord. As in Lyme disease, the syphilis spirochete enters the nervous system during the early-disseminated phase, when spirochetes travel in the bloodstream. Also as in Lyme disease, these spirochetes may cause no symptoms at all, or they can produce a usually mild case of meningitis.

Late syphilis of the central nervous system primarily caused two syndromes—general paresis and tabes dorsalis. The former—which caused paranoia, emotional instability, delusions, and hallucinations as well as problems with memory, judgment, and insight—was a serious public health problem during the nineteenth and early twentieth centuries. The latter caused spinal cord damage. Lack of effective treatment of the early stages of syphilis led to huge numbers patients with these later manifestations. In 1921, it was estimated that 10 percent of all patients in British mental institutions were victims of general paresis, "and most of them were destined to die a wretched, lingering death," according to one source. During this time, of the 1,559 patients admitted with general paresis to St. Elizabeth's Hospital in Washington, D.C., 77 percent died from the disease. In another review of 1,500 untreated cases, the mortality was 80 percent. Most of these deaths occurred within four years of diagnosis.

Because the principal symptoms were psychiatric, psychiatrists usually treated these patients. At the time, mercury rubs were used, which often resulted in more of a toxic than therapeutic response, but this therapy was still mentioned as useful in early syphilis in the seventh edition of Osler's famous textbook *Principles and Practice of*

Medicine, published in 1909: "A drachm of the ordinary mercurial ointment is thoroughly rubbed into the skin every evening for six days; on the seventh, a warm bath is taken, and on the eighth the mercurial course is resumed." Of general paresis, however, Osler wrote, "Careful nursing and the orderly life of an asylum are the only measures necessary in a great majority of the cases."

The syphilis spirochete, *T. pallidum,* was discovered in 1905. In 1909, German microbiologist Paul Ehrlich (after whom the genus *Ehrlichia* is named) methodically sought out the "magic bullet" that would kill the microorganism but leave the human host unharmed. He used arsenic derivatives, meticulously testing compound after compound on laboratory animals experimentally infected with *T. pallidum.* After more than six hundred tries, he found salvarsan (arsphenamine) and later the improved neosalvarsan (neoarsphenamine). In 1908, Ehrlich was awarded the Nobel Prize in medicine for his work on antimicrobial chemotherapy.

Although these arsenic compounds were of some value in treating early syphilis, they both produced frequent side effects. More importantly, neither worked particularly well in late-stage neurosyphilis. Thus, general paresis remained a serious problem. Wrote one expert as late as 1929, general paresis is "perhaps the most terrible of all mankind's diseases and . . . its diagnosis has been accepted as a sentence of death, to take effect at the latest within four years, generally much sooner."

As early as 1887, Austrian psychiatrist Julius Wagner von Jauregg began his work on treating patients with late-stage syphilis and was intrigued by the idea of using fever as a cure. He wrote in his 1922 paper "The Treatment of General Paresis by Inoculation of Malaria": "We could scarcely speak of a treatment of general paresis and tabes which had recovery in view before the knowledge of the syphilitic etiology of these diseases had been established. . . . We began to treat this disease antisyphilitically after the [syphilitic] nature of general paresis became known, first with the old means—mercury and iodides—later with salvarsan. Neither the old nor the new treatment of syphilis could boast of special results in regard to general paresis. Not that temporary improvement was not to be reached in that way in individual cases. The advance of the disease could be checked for a longer period especially through salvarsan. But the remissions were rarely complete and never lasting. The movement came finally, whether earlier or later, in which the fatal tragedy could no longer be warded off from the patient.

"The discovery that not rarely psychoses were healed through intercurrent infectious diseases instigated me already in 1887 to the proposal that one should intentionally imitate this experiment of nature for the cure of psychoses. And already at this time, I mentioned malaria as one of the diseases suitable for this. It can be artificially produced, is not too dangerous for the patient and his environment and in each case, can be interrupted again."

Wagner von Jauregg tried other means of producing fevers. He first tried the tuberculin preparation that Robert Koch had made from the tuberculosis bacillus. Next he experimented with a typhus vaccine. Finally he settled on induced malaria. The technique was to draw a few milliliters of blood from a malaria-infected donor and then inject this infected blood under the skin beneath the shoulder blade of the patient infected with late-stage syphilis. Larger "doses" of malarious blood would reduce the incubation period from two weeks to just a few days.

In the summer of 1917 he inoculated nine syphilitic patients with malaria and had a "plainly favorable" response in six of the nine. He made further experiments in 1919 and then began to use the method continuously. Wagner von Jauregg successfully treated patients whose neurosyphilis manifested as dementia, mania, delirium, and delusions of grandeur. "Complete remission occurred in more than 50 of the paretics selected for treatment so far," he wrote. "They were not only capable of taking up their occupations but for the most part are actually at work at their former calling. This result is so much more gratifying since so far, a return of the condition has not occurred in a single one of these completely remitted cases."

Wagner von Jauregg concluded his paper by noting: "Above all one must see to it that the paretics are brought to treatment in the earliest stages possible. This is the most important condition upon which the result depends."

The mortality rate from the therapy (that is, from the malaria itself) was low. In one investigator's experience with 1,600 cases treated with malariatherapy, it was below 2 percent. The mortality rate of patients with general paresis treated with malariatherapy dropped from upward of 70 percent to below 10 percent. So enormous was the burden of late-stage neurosyphilis at the time and so dramatic was the cure rate that Wagner von Jauregg was awarded the Nobel Prize in medicine in 1927 for his work. These days, of course, malariatherapy is no longer used to treat neurosyphilis as antibiotics were developed that could cure it more quickly, easily, safely, and effectively.

When Mary Walker's father got her phone call, he didn't know any of this. Although he was "appalled" by her idea of malariatherapy, he quickly decided that "it was best to help her rather than to have her attempt it on her own. In the succeeding days I spoke with microbiologists, parasitologists, physicians, and scientists in our country, as well as in England, Sweden, Canada, Mexico, and Costa Rica. I came to the conclusion that there was a chance that it might work."

He and Mary went to Belize, hoping she would be able to contract malaria naturally by mosquito bite. Traveling to a remote village by British Army Land Rover, the Walkers arrived at a group of thatched huts populated by El Salvadoran refugees. After spending the night in one such mud-floored hut devoid of furniture, they passed time by the river. "The best mosquito exposure was along the river, although there were quite a few right in the hut," Walker recalls. "By the time Mary had received over 200 bites (perhaps nearer 300) she was pretty uncomfortable. I decided that we should return to the United States rather than wait in Belize during the incubation period. Conditions are quite primitive in Belize, and I wanted to avoid needing medical care there." Unfortunately, despite these hundreds of bites, Mary did not become infected.

Next, the Walkers traveled to Mexico, where a professor of parasitology helped them obtain blood from a child infected with active malaria. Receiving blood from a patient with malaria increased the chances of becoming infected, but also increased the risks of getting other blood-borne infections. The child's blood was tested for HIV, hepatitis, and other infectious diseases before being injected into Mary's vein, but although these precautions diminished the risk, they did not negate it. After Mary received five milliliters of blood, the Walkers again returned to the United States, but again, she did not develop malaria.

Yet again the Walkers returned to Mexico City where Mary received another injection of blood from a pediatric malaria patient. This time, the doctor with whom they were working met them at the airport in an ambulance. After Mary received the injection in the ambulance, the Walkers flew directly back to the States. Eighteen days later, Mary started running a fever, accompanied by vomiting and chills. The fever, which was allowed to persist for ninety-six hours, raged as high as 106 degrees, and Mary's pulse rocketed to as high as 150 beats per minute. When her spleen became enlarged, her father initiated treatment for the malaria.

Unfortunately, the original symptoms of Lyme disease persisted, so they repeated the entire procedure still another time. During this next course of malaria, Mary endured 136 hours of fever. Again, however, her original symptoms persisted. In the end, the Walkers concluded that the malariatherapy was a failure.

How could malaria, or other infectious diseases as observed by Wagner von Jauregg, cure syphilis or Lyme disease? Was it simply the heat of the fever? If so, surely a person's body temperature could be artificially raised without resorting to the risks of acquiring malaria or being injected with someone else's blood. In the 1920s, some physicians tried heating devices, the most popular being the Electronic Cabinet of Kettering, named for the General Motors engineer who also invented the electronic ignition for automobiles. Nonetheless, heat alone was generally thought to be inferior to induced malaria. Malariatherapy is thought to work not only from the physical rise in temperature, but also from the other immunostimulative effects that malaria causes in humans. Patients with malaria generate higher levels of interleukins and interferons—infection-fighting substances that are not specific antibodies to a particular organism.

As recently as 1996, European investigators reported that high temperatures can inhibit the growth of *B. burgdorferi* and that the effect of antibiotics with high temperature was additive. It was also found that the ability of *B. burgdorferi* to grow at various temperatures was at least partly a function of strain; some strains possess a greater ability to grow at higher temperatures than others.

While some continue this line of research—including Dr. Heimlich, who has suggested that malariatherapy could be useful in treating patients infected with HIV—malariatherapy is not endorsed by the CDC, the conventional camp, or the alternative camp for the treatment of Lyme disease. Isolated physicians have tried it, and other physicians have helped their patients who made their own decisions to use malariatherapy in the same spirit that Walker helped his daughter. In this regard, Walker makes an important point when he says: "It is very easy for healthy people to criticize the desperate actions of those who are so ill. But only those who are suffering can know the desperation that drives people to take radical chances to get well."

24 • Genomes and Vaccines

Given all the controversy over therapy, hopes ran high that continued work on both the genetic structure of *B. burgdorferi* and the development of a vaccine would lead to better preventive strategies, diagnostic tests, and treatments for Lyme disease.

By the closing decade of the twentieth century, molecular biology had evolved to levels that only could have been dreamt of fifty years ago when scientists discovered the structure of DNA. DNA was discovered in the late 1860s and had been known to carry genetic information since the 1940s. Found inside all living cells, DNA is composed of smaller components, bases called purines and pyrimidines. In fact, just four of these compounds comprise DNA—two purines (adenine and guanine) and two pyrimidines (thymine and cytosine). At the mid-century mark, the additional finding that DNA always contained a one-to-one ratio of adenine to thymine and of guanine to cytosine was made; the bases seemed to be paired. The molecular structure of DNA, however, remained obscure.

In 1953, armed with this information, as well as healthy doses of curiosity and youthful hubris, James Watson and Francis Crick began working on that structure at Cambridge University in England.

After many false starts, they finally proposed the structure of DNA—that of a double helix consisting of two strands, each acting as a template for the other. In April 1953, they wrote in the journal *Nature,* "It has not escaped our notice that the specific pairing [of bases] we have postulated immediately suggests a possible copying mechanism for the genetic material."

Their double helix fit all the data. Adenine and guanine in one strand always bound to thymine and cytosine, respectively, in the other, thus accounting for the base pairing. The helical structure, which could come apart and regenerate, provided a copying mechanism for passing genetic information from one generation to the next.

Their finding became the building block for numerous scientific advances over the next fifty years and is considered by some to be the most important scientific discovery of the twentieth century. It was a necessary precursor to molecular biology that today we almost take for granted. Work with DNA, as we have already seen, led to the development of the technique of PCR, so useful for the diagnosis of many infectious diseases.

With an understanding of DNA and the development of techniques to tease it apart, scientists could decode the entire genetic structure of *B. burgdorferi.* And that is precisely what they did. A team spearheaded by Claire Fraser, president and director of The Institute for Genomic Research, undertook the task of defining the genome, or entire genetic structure, of *B. burgdorferi.* Other microbes had been already selected for this kind of analysis, and Fraser's group wanted to choose an important microbe and something from the unique spirochete family. The process, says Fraser, "is fairly straightforward. First you isolate the DNA using standard methods, purify it, then physically break it up into small pieces." She then continues, as if rattling off the recipe to cook a stew. The pieces of DNA are cloned and made into plasmids, bits of genetic material that can then be inserted into the bacterium *E. coli.* The *E. coli,* as it multiplies, which it does frenetically, acts as a little manufacturing plant, pumping out vast quantities of the plasmid, until finally, there is sufficient quantity to work with. Essentially, each plasmid is a random piece of the DNA of *B. burgdorferi.*

Knowing the general size of the genome of the spirochete, the scientists generate enough different plasmids until they have made approximately eight times the entire genome. This kind of redundancy helps to ensure that they have the entire genome.

Enter computers. Using programs of enormous complexity, computers sequence the base pairs—that is, they determine the sequence, or order, of the pairs of adenine and thymine or guanine and cytosine. Each base pair is stained with a different fluorescent dye, which is then read by a laser that feeds the information into the computer. The machine spits out the base pair sequence. "Then it becomes like putting a jigsaw puzzle together," notes Fraser. The computer reads the sequence of the next two base pairs, the next four base pairs, the next eight base pairs, and so on. It searches out these sequences, looking for overlap of specific base pair sequences. These overlap regions are like the corner pieces in the puzzle and allow the computer to "orient" itself and to know when to stop; the computer will continue sequencing until there is no overlap left. There are no new sequences. The program will run again and again to make sure that there are no duplicate pieces.

Next the scientists will check for duplicate "pieces" of base pairs and use some other techniques, including PCR, to fill in any perceived gaps. At this point, it is relatively easy to delineate the microbial genes, since most bacteria are "wall-to-wall genes," says Fraser. Molecular biologists know certain start and stop sequences (sequences that mark the boundaries of individual genes) because these tend to be well-conserved, or used over and over again, in different biological species, not only in bacteria but in higher cells as well. The fact that these base pair sequences are conserved illustrates their biological importance, in a Darwinian sense, that is, in the sense that they have withstood millions of years of evolutionary pressure and remain nature's solution to a particular problem. Fraser and colleagues found that the genome of *B. burgdorferi* contains one linear chromosome of nearly one million base pairs and at least twenty-one plasmids whose combined number of base pairs number over half a million. One of the interesting findings was that many of the genes, especially those based on the plasmids, had no known biological function although the researchers speculated that they were related to antigenic variation and immune evasion. This means that *B. burgdorferi* can change its outer appearance to the immune system—a good strategy from the perspective of the spirochete.

Why is it important to know the genetic structure of an organism? Says Fraser, "Once you've got the genome, you've got a 'parts list' of the organism. Because of the high degree of conserved DNA across many types of cells, one can infer, to some degree, the function of many genes," which helps scientists better understand an organism. Of course one does not know everything about what a gene does solely on the basis of its structure, but that knowledge frequently allows for intelligent guesses. Working with information about other organisms, biologists know when a protein is membrane bound (it has many hydrophobic amino acids that anchor it in the membrane and tend to form alpha helixes, a common protein structure) or when they code for a protein that is destined to be secreted (they know the signal sequences for secretion) from a cell.

Understanding an organism's genome is only the first small step in understanding the organism; it opens the door to a huge amount of potential work. Fraser offers the analogy that working with an organism whose genome is known versus unknown is akin to working with the lights on versus off. Fraser and her team of nearly forty colleagues published their work in the December 1997 issue of *Nature*. It may take several more years to reap the benefits of this work.

Some initial findings are of historical interest. For one, recall Dr. Richard Kelly's finding the right culture medium to grow borreliae (see Chapter 12). He needed to tinker with the ingredients by adding *N*-acetylglucosamine. Fraser was able to make sense of that finding by identifying an *N*-acetylglucosamine transport system that would allow the spirochete to import that substance into its internal milieu.

This is the kind of finding—a new transport protein, or a particular growth requirement—that could open a door to a new therapeutic discovery. If *B. burgdorferi* has a unique membrane transport system that could be blocked, a substance might be found to block it, which could lead to new drug therapies. If *B. burgdorferi* were found to have a novel growth requirement, a better diagnostic test might possibly be developed. Similarly, as we learn more about borreliae in general, it is possible that findings will allow scientists to culture organisms that currently cannot be cultivated—such as the presumed bacterium causing the Lyme-like disease that Masters and colleagues are seeing across the southern United States. Newer vaccines could also be developed from information that comes from knowing the genome.

One example of the potential clinical payoff in this basic science is with regards to *Neisseria meningitidis*—the bacterium that causes the most severe form of meningitis. Italian scientists, led by M. Pizza, were working on problems with a vaccine for *N. meningitidis*—finding a protein that had specific characteristics. The candidate protein needed to be surface-exposed (on the bacteria's outer surface), not cross-react with human proteins, and exhibit little sequence variation. Knowing the genome of the bacterium allowed Pizza's group to create and test properties of more than 350 candidate proteins for those properties known to correlate with vaccine effectiveness in humans.

The Institute for Genomic Research is also examining the genomes of other spirochetes, searching for both similarities and differences between them and *B. burgdorferi*. Conserved genes are presumably more important inasmuch as they have survived the Darwinian test of evolutionary pressure.

During the 1990s, other researchers began to test a vaccine for Lyme disease. The concept of creating a vaccine to prevent a disease came two centuries before the explosion of molecular biology in relation to a disease thought to be eradicated from the planet in 1979—smallpox. Even as we enter this new millennium, however, doubt has been cast on how complete that eradication has truly been. Once again, the United States is massing a huge inventory of smallpox vaccine.

Most schoolchildren learn about the British physician Edward Jenner, who pioneered the concept of vaccination. A country doctor, Jenner practiced in the small village of Berkeley in Gloucestershire. Most schoolchildren, however, will not have heard about Lady Mary Wortley Montagu, the wife of the British ambassador to the Turkish court. In 1718, Lady Montagu had her three-year-old son inoculated against smallpox, which at that time had overtaken the plague as the number one killer in England. Lady Montagu, a member of the London upper class, was in Istanbul when she herself was stricken by smallpox. Although she survived, she was left with severe facial scarring, which greatly affected her beauty. Wishing to avoid her son getting ill, she had him undergo the procedure of inoculation, a method that was popular in the Arab world and which Montagu wrote was called engrafting. "Every year, thousands undergo this operation," she wrote, "and the French Ambassador says pleasantly, that they take the small-pox here by way of diversion, as they take the waters in other countries. . . . I am patriot enough to take the pains to bring this useful invention into fashion in England, and I should not fail to write to some of our doctors very particularly about it, if I knew any one of them that I thought had virtue enough to destroy such a considerable branch of their revenue, for the good of mankind."

The procedure consisted of placing a small amount of material from an active pox of a smallpox patient into an open cut of the person receiving the inoculation. Although there was no real scientific basis for the procedure, it seemed to work in some people, who would get a mild case of smallpox but be left immune to serious disease. Roughly 12 percent of people who were inoculated died; however, nearly 30 percent of people who got smallpox died. Despite Lady Montagu's public relations campaign to popularize the practice, it was never fully embraced. Nevertheless, some physicians used the method, including Jenner.

But Jenner had problems persuading some of the locals in Berkeley to be inoculated. Jenner worked in the countryside, where many people worked with cows and many of those got cowpox, an infection that affected cattle but could also infect humans, producing blisters where their hands touched the cows' udders. The disease was never fatal to humans, and local folklore held that a bout of cowpox would leave that person forever immune to smallpox.

Like Mrs. Mensch and Mrs. Murray, the townspeople had been living a reality different from that of local physicians. And like Steere, Jenner had the wisdom to observe and study a new idea. He found

that the local milkmaids were correct—cowpox patients became immune to subsequent attack by smallpox. The power of these observations take on even more significance when it is remembered that all
of this occurred in the mid-eighteenth century, long before scientists
knew of bacteria, let alone the much smaller viruses that caused these
two poxes

On May 14, 1796, the country doctor performed an experiment
that would forever change the medical world. He scraped some of
the fluid from the lesion on the arm of a milkmaid who had cowpox
and placed it into the fresh cut on a young boy named James Phipps.
Eight days later, the boy developed cowpox and then recovered. Six
weeks later, Jenner purposefully placed some material from a smallpox patient into cuts on the boy's arm. Young Phipps never contracted smallpox. Jenner performed the same experiment on twenty-
three other people; none fell ill with smallpox. He concluded that
people who had had cowpox became immune to smallpox. He named
the process *vaccination* (from the Latin word for cow—*vacca*) to distinguish it from inoculation.

Jenner's manuscripts were initially rejected for publication, and
finally he self-published his work in 1798. Over the next several years,
vaccination for smallpox became increasingly popular and accepted
by the medical establishment, but not without more bumps in the
road. Some tried to take credit for Jenner's work. Others condemned
it, claiming that intentionally infecting people with cowpox was unethical and would create other serious medical problems. Nevertheless, fewer than two hundred years later, naturally acquired smallpox
had been wiped off the face of the earth.

Louis Pasteur, a French chemist, made the next great stride in
the field of vaccinations. The European wine and beer industries per-
suaded Pasteur to develop techniques to prevent spoilage in their
products. After doing so (inventing the technique of *pasteurization*),
the European poultry industry called upon Pasteur in 1871. Their
flocks of chickens and turkeys were being decimated by an infection
called chicken cholera that was spreading from farm to farm. Using
the meticulous experimental technique for which he was known,
Pasteur discovered that he could vaccinate chickens with old, weak-

ened bacteria and prevent the disease. Single-handedly, he saved the poultry industry. Next, he extended these findings to anthrax, another disease that has surfaced in our era with its renewed fears of bio-terrorism.

Pasteur found that if he inactivated the anthrax bacillus that Robert Koch had isolated, he could use it to vaccinate animals and prevent them from becoming infected. His successes led to his work on a vaccine for rabies, a uniformly fatal disease in humans that was transmitted by the bite of a rabid animal. After hundreds of animal experiments, Pasteur succeeded in finding a vaccine that worked in dogs. Before he had begun testing on humans, a frantic mother begged Pasteur to try the vaccine on her nine-year-old son, who had been bitten by a rabid wolf. Again, Pasteur prevailed; he used the vaccine and the boy lived.

Over the next century, doctors' work with vaccines gradually improved their effectiveness and expanded the number of diseases for which vaccines were available. Medicine and immunology finally caught up with the dramatic findings of Jenner, Pasteur, and others.

Recall that in testing for *B. burgdorferi*, the various tests measure for antibodies, proteins manufactured against antigens by immune cells in mammals. The antigens are foreign-shaped proteins that create the surface texture of various microorganisms. In the case of smallpox and cowpox, the surface shapes of these two related viruses are sufficiently similar so that antibodies formed to the cowpox virus will also attack the smallpox virus. After little James Phipps developed cowpox, some of his lymphocytes manufactured antibodies that would attack the cowpox virus. Six weeks later, when he was challenged with smallpox, his lymphocytes recognized the same shape and had a running start at making antibodies that would kill the smallpox virus, thinking that it was another bout of cowpox.

Pasteur's vaccine for chicken cholera worked by injecting a weakened strain of the bacterium. Not powerful enough to cause the disease, the bacterium still retained enough of its surface shape and texture so that the chickens' immune system made antibodies against it. If a bird was subsequently exposed to the virulent strain of the cholera bacillus, its lymphocytes stood primed and ready to start making antibodies that would kill the cholera bug before it could do any damage. Pasteur's anthrax vaccine worked in the same way, except instead of using a weakened but live vaccine, he inactivated the anthrax with a powerful chemical called phenol. Nevertheless, the recipient animal's immune system recognized the shape and made antibodies so if the virulent anthrax bacillus ever infected that animal, the body would mount an antibody response and repel the infection.

It was only a matter of time before doctors would try to find a vaccine for Lyme disease. In their search they hoped to find some piece of the outer surface of *B. burgdorferi* that after injection into a patient would be recognized by that person's immune system and provoke an antibody response. Then, if an infected tick ever bit that same person, the antibodies would kill the spirochete before it did any damage.

Work during the latter half of the 1980s led to the characterization of the various outer surface proteins, labeled Osp A, Osp B, Osp C, and so forth. Using the techniques of molecular biology, researchers could insert the genes for making these proteins into *E. coli* bacteria that would then manufacture the proteins. In the early 1990s, one of these proteins, Osp A, was tested. When injected into mice, it induced them to develop antibodies to the protein, and then these mice could not be infected with *B. burgdorferi*. Next, doctors performed preliminary tests on humans. This work, published in 1994, found that the vaccine did induce an antibody response in humans and was safe.

These findings were expanded by work done through the mid-1990s, and large-scale human trials were started. In the July 23, 1998, issue of the *New England Journal of Medicine*, two studies were published. One was directed by Dr. Steere and tested the product made by SmithKline Beecham Pharmaceuticals. The other was directed by Dr. Leonard Sigal and tested a similar product made by Connaught. Both products used Osp A vaccines. The data from both studies were similar and showed that the vaccines prevented Lyme disease, but only in about 80 percent of the subjects. Eighty percent protection is not bad, but it is a lot less than the efficacy for most vaccines, which falls closer to 97 or 98 percent.

One aspect of both vaccines was quite unique. Every human vaccine to this point had worked by producing antibodies that kill the invading organism in the bloodstream or extracellular tissues of the human. The Lyme vaccine, in theory, was different. The antibodies that were produced in the bloodstream were sucked by the biting tick and actually killed the spirochetes in the *tick's* body rather than the human's body.

The two drug companies raced to see which could bring the vaccine to market first. Surely a preventive vaccine would provide common ground for all the participants in the Lyme debate. Such was not the case, however. During the initial hearings of the Food and Drug Administration (FDA) in May 1998, some concerns were expressed about the theoretical possibility of side effects from an Osp A vaccination. Some patients with chronic antibiotic-resistant Lyme arthritis had very high levels of antibodies to Osp A; many of these patients had a certain gene called DR4, a gene that approximately 30 percent of the general population carry. There were concerns that this segment of the population might develop side effects to the vaccine. SmithKline Beecham assured the FDA and the advisory board that this was not the case, but promised more research.

Dr. Patricia Ferrieri chaired the advisory board and noted that "It's rare that a vaccine is voted on with such ambivalence and such a stack of provisos." Despite these concerns, in December 1998 the FDA licensed the SmithKline Beecham product, called LYMErix. As has been true for nearly every breakthrough on Lyme disease, however, the controversy over the Osp A vaccine has not only persisted, it has intensified.

25 • Legal and Political Battles

After the release of any new vaccine or drug on the market, scientists, epidemiologists, physicians, the government, and the manufacturer of the vaccine look for side effects. This process is called *post-marketing surveillance* and is vitally important even though the initial FDA-required studies, known as phase three studies, have already shown that a drug or vaccine is likely safe. Phase three studies, however, examine hundreds or thousands of patients, rather than tens or hundreds of thousands. From time to time, a drug or vaccine comes out that looks good in the phase three studies but proves to be dangerous when it is used in larger numbers of individuals.

Post-marketing surveillance also is important because it will show the effects that exist during routine use of the product in the community, not merely the investigational use in the closely monitored context of a scientific study. Furthermore, side effects that might not have been identified simply because of the study design and definitions will often emerge during post-marketing surveillance.

As a part of the original trials of LYMErix, SmithKline Beecham looked for adverse effects in several ways. For one, immediately after vaccination, a subset of vaccinees was given a four-day diary card on which they recorded any unusual reactions. Second, the study involved six follow-up visits, during which adverse effects could be recorded. As well, at month twenty, a safety postcard was mailed to vaccinees to remind them to report any vaccine-related problems. As in any scientific trial of a vaccine, a data safety monitoring board was in place to review the data coming in.

All of this sounds very thorough; surely such a net would capture any side effects the vaccine caused. However, there is lively debate on this issue. According to the company, now called GlaxoSmithKline, there was no evidence that the vaccine was dangerous. The company found no lack of safety in analyzing the diary cards, the symptoms reported at the follow-up visits, and the twenty-month follow-up safety postcards. It looked at patients who had had prior Lyme disease and reported no significant increase in persistent adverse effects in the vaccinated group compared with the placebo group (those patients in the study who received a dummy injection).

Regarding the patients who carry the DR4 gene, the company pointed out that 30 percent of the population carries this gene and that although it did not specifically analyze DR4-positive patients in its large studies, these patients were represented just by their frequency in the general population. Furthermore, the company did some studies on rodents that suggested that the Osp A vaccine did not cause arthritis in these experimental animals.

Nevertheless, reports of adverse effects associated with LYMErix began to surface. Patients began complaining to their doctors that they developed joint problems after the vaccine; they also began reporting various neurological and pain syndromes. For the most part, these patients were healthy before being vaccinated, as one might expect, as those who elected to be vaccinated generally spent significant periods of time outdoors.

On January 31, 2001, the FDA held public hearings on LYMErix to reassess the vaccine. Dr. Robert Ball presented information about yet another way that the government monitors for vaccine side effects. This system is the vaccine adverse effects reporting system, known as VAERS. Jointly managed by the FDA and CDC, VAERS is a national system for surveillance of adverse events after vaccination. It receives about eleven thousand reports of adverse events per year—from physicians, manufacturers, and patients. This casts a wide net of surveillance, but not one without gaps. Many of the diagnoses cannot be verified because of the lack of medical records or consistent diagnostic coding. As for Lyme disease, there is acknowledged underreporting.

Furthermore, the denominator—that is, the number of doses of vaccine actually administered—is unknown. Even though the manufacturer reports the number of vaccine doses that have been distributed, it is unknown how many have actually been injected into patients. This is important with LYMErix. Although 1.4 million doses have been distributed, it simply cannot be known how many of those doses are sitting on shelves in physician's offices or clinics. As well, most patients receive three doses of vaccine, so even if all 1.4 million doses were given, the number of patients would be about only 450,000. The rate of adverse events is the number of events (the numerator) divided by the number of patients who receive the vaccine (the denominator). Since neither number is known with precision, their ratio cannot be accurately calculated.

"Perhaps the biggest limitation," according to Ned Hayes, chief of the epidemiology section of the CDC's bacterial zoonoses division, "is that VAERS is a passive surveillance system." The passive system waits for results to come to it, as opposed to the active system, which goes out and looks for problems. Despite all this, Hayes feels that most of the side effects would be counted because LYMErix was a new product, a lot of publicity surrounded it, and physicians were encouraged to report problems. "However," he cautioned, "we have no way to know what percentage of adverse effects was actually reported."

With its limitations, however, VAERS is the system we have. Ball reported on nearly two years of VAERS data on LYMErix that showed 1,048 reports of problems. These included 4 deaths and 85 "serious reactions" (defined as leading to hospitalization, prolongation of a hospital stay, or development of disability or a life-threatening illness). It is important to note that these reports do not necessarily imply a causal relationship to the vaccine, only a temporal one. For example, someone could get a dose of a vaccine and then have a heart attack twelve hours later, but this does not mean that the vaccine caused the heart attack. It is also important to know that most adverse effects associated with a vaccine are trivial—some soreness or redness at the injection site, a bit of muscle discomfort, or low-grade fever for a day or so afterward.

The FDA personnel who analyze these reports do what epidemiologists do: they look for commonality. They look for clustering of a lag time from vaccination to side effect, for similarity in the symptoms and gender of patients affected. They planned to interview two hundred of the patients, but by the FDA hearings in January 2001, they had spoken to only thirty-five of them.

GlaxoSmithKline was also conducting a phase four study—a post-marketing study to look for side effects in the larger community population. The original SmithKline Beecham trial vaccinated about five thousand patients; the planned phase four study targeted twenty-five thousand.

To the FDA's credit, it allowed private citizens to testify at the advisory committee meeting. Some testified that they had developed severe pain syndromes, arthritis, and even an unusual form of spinal cord inflammation called transverse myelitis. Karen Forschner expressed numerous concerns, saying: "We have concern over the scientific evidence and criteria being not completely scrutinized and published. We are concerned about the closed loop and difficulty of other opinions and scientists getting into these government discussions and looking at the data. We are concerned about conflict of interest. . . . We are concerned about informed consents to patients both with prior Lyme and on the HAL [DR4] issue." Concerning adverse effects of the vaccine, she said, "We are concerned that the data that was captured before is still the same data that you are capturing now, and may not actually represent what is actually happening to patients in the real world. We are concerned about the definitions used for vaccine failures."

Dr. Sidney Wolfe of the Public Citizen's Health Research Group compared the issues that were in play with LYMErix to those that surrounded the swine flu vaccine debacle in the late 1970s, which resulted in an outbreak of Guillain-Barré syndrome, another inflammatory problem of the nervous system. Wolfe also formally objected to the company's "reckless promotion" of the vaccine to the public through advertising. During these January 2001 hearings, there were various calls to modify the package insert of the vaccine (which gives instructions to health-care workers about risks), to change the informed consent of patients receiving the vaccine, to send out an informational letter to all physicians, and even to suspend use of the vaccine. However, the FDA's radar did not show cause for alarm, and it elected to take none of these actions.

Changing course on a vaccine is not unknown; in fact, during the same time, the FDA pulled a vaccine that it had recently deemed safe and effective. On August 31, 1998, the federal agency licensed a vaccine against rotavirus for use in infants. Rotavirus is a common cause of childhood gastroenteritis that leads to diarrhea, vomiting, and abdominal cramps. In the United States, it results in a few dozen deaths each year, but worldwide, rotavirus accounts for an estimated six hundred thousand deaths annually among infants and toddlers. Thus, the vaccine has important public health implications.

The Advisory Committee on Immunization Practices, the American Academy of Pediatrics, and the American Academy of Family Physicians recommended its routine use in healthy infants. During the safety trials conducted by Wyeth-Lederle, five infants developed intussusception, a serious condition in which one portion of the intestine telescopes onto another, causing bleeding and bowel obstruction and sometimes requiring surgical repair. The five cases of intussusception occurred among 10,054 vaccine recipients and one of 4,633 control subjects, a difference that was not statistically significant.

In the ten months after licensure, fifteen cases of intussusception among infants who had received the rotavirus vaccine were reported to VAERS. Half of them required surgery. As well, a phase four study done in California also concluded that vaccinees had an increased risk of intussusception. Although the FDA did not consider the phase four study or the VAERS findings conclusive, they recommended a moratorium on use of the rotavirus vaccine; the various academies pulled their recommendation as well. In October 1999, just a year after it was approved, the vaccine was delicensed.

At the January 2001 FDA hearings concerning LYMErix, Dr.

Ferrieri, who had expressed some concerns at the May 1998 meeting (which resulted in approval), had accumulated even more doubts. "My concern is greater than it was before," she said, "and there are several areas that we have not yet been able to gain information on that I commented on before . . . the issue of further boosters, the length of protection, etc. In a nutshell, I think FDA has to grapple with the serious issue of [whether] it is sufficient to do revisions to the package insert." Addressing two FDA officials present at the meeting, she asked, "How far will you be pushed to have to do something more drastic than that?"

Ferrieri emphasized her feeling that she had never before heard such concerns expressed "without Agency response that has satisfied the dissatisfying from my point of view. I consider what we're dealing with today to be very, very serious, and I would like to throw back to you the need for you all to reexamine how this fits in to your mission and in the public health realm."

Others on the panel expressed doubts and disappointment as well, but in the end, the FDA elected not to make any changes—no changes to the package insert, no moratorium, and certainly no pulling of the license.

The FDA vaccine advisory committee met again on November 28, 2001, to discuss the Lyme disease vaccine. Forschner of the Lyme Disease Foundation again testified, and like Ferrieri, she was more concerned than ever. "Based on the new data I am presenting today," she said, "I believe that the Osp A vaccine represents an imminent and substantial hazard to the public health and needs to be immediately recalled." Using more than ten exhibits to make her points, Forschner called the Lyme vaccine process "seriously flawed" and charged that information had been withheld from both the committee and the FDA in such a way as to "compromise all trial data and even cast doubt on the integrity of the investigators."

Representing many of the people who assert that they have been harmed by the vaccine is Stephen Sheller, a Philadelphia lawyer, whose firm launched a class action suit against the manufacturer at the end of 1999. Sheller became involved in an unusual way. "I was contacted by a law firm representing a large group of physicians who were concerned that the vaccine was extremely dangerous," recalls Sheller. "They also believed that the vaccine effectiveness was doubtful at best and that the trials were potentially compromised by conflicts of interest. They were also concerned that many physicians would end up as defendants on medical malpractice cases as the adverse events accumulated." So Sheller met in his office with these doctors "who were trying their best to protect public health."

Another interesting phenomenon related to the vaccine was the manufacturer's assertion that vaccine use did not affect the ability of blood tests to detect Lyme disease in vaccine recipients. Although the vaccine would make the ELISA positive, it should not affect the Western blot, the test that could distinguish between different specific antibodies to *B. burgdorferi*. More than one investigator, however, found that the vaccine did affect the Western blot—and not just in the Osp A area; the vaccine seemed to induce several antibodies that made the blot impossible to properly interpret.

Dr. Paul Fawcett, the Delaware immunologist and Lyme serology expert, found that patients who received the Osp A vaccine not only developed an antibody band at the Osp A region on the Western blot test strip, but some vaccine recipients also made many other bands. Using one commercial test kit, he found so many antibody bands that tests were positive even using the Dearborn criteria. In a paper that he and colleagues published in January 2001, he concluded, "The usefulness of all three Western blot assays for the diagnosis of potential infection in a vaccine recipient is severely limited by the extensive reactivity caused by vaccination alone." Even more significant, Fawcett and his colleagues published a clinical account of four patients—two children and two adults—who developed arthritis after vaccination with LYMErix. The pattern of arthritis—a polyarthritis involving multiple small joints—was atypical for naturally acquired Lyme arthritis, which usually is an oligoarticular process involving just a few large joints (generally the knees).

Despite all of these bits of information, as of early February 2002, the FDA had not taken any action regarding LYMErix.

It is worth noting that these regulatory issues are not unique to Lyme disease. For instance, class action suits were filed against the

German industrial giant Bayer when its cholesterol-lowering drug Baycol was found to cause deaths from destruction of muscle tissue. The original number of deaths was small, and then was estimated at fifty-two, only to be revised upward to one hundred, according to a Reuters Medical News report in early 2002. The FDA initially licensed this drug but later withdrew that license.

The May 19, 2001, issue of the British medical journal *Lancet* contained an editorial titled "Lotronex and the FDA: A Fatal Erosion of Integrity." In this piece, Richard Horton takes the FDA to task for its too close association with GlaxoSmithKline regarding the licensing and promotion of a new drug, Lotronex, marketed for irritable bowel syndrome. According to Horton, there were clear-cut signs that some patients were experiencing a serious and potentially fatal side effect. "Instead of withdrawing Lotronex and calling for more evidence," Horton writes, "the FDA issued a medication guide designed to warn patients of escalating risks, while keeping the drug on the market. This decision was to prove fatal. On November 28, GlaxoWelcome withdrew Lotronex from the market after the deaths of five patients taking the drug. . . . In addition to the deaths, 24 patients had required admission to hospital and 10 needed surgery." This was another case in which there was some question of a problem before approval, and as with LYMErix, the company was to do some post-marketing studies.

Responses from the FDA were published in the August 4, 2001, issue of *Lancet,* but Horton stood his ground, reporting on the results of an internal inquiry by the FDA's Center for Drug Evaluation and Research. Its own survey showed that "reviewers complained not only of 'editing' of reviews by team leaders, deputy division directors and division directors, but also of 'requests' to change their opinions. Reviewers reported 'pressure to favor the desires of sponsors [drug companies] over science and the public health.' The report notes that 'one third of our respondents did not feel comfortable expressing their differing scientific opinion.' Moreover, reviewers argued that 'decisions should be based more on science and less on corporate wishes.' Too often, decisions that went against the company 'are stigmatized in the Agency.' One of the 13 recommendations in the report is to 'encourage freedom of expression of scientific opinion.'"

An external survey of FDA medical officers who handle new drug applications drew similar conclusions.

Given the controversies surrounding Lyme disease and its vaccine, it is not surprising that Lyme disease made its way into the courtroom as well. New York lawyer Ira Maurer tried one of the first cases in 1993, representing some railroad workers who maintained that they had developed Lyme disease because of their occupation. Maurer prevailed in that case and began to represent others with Lyme disease. "Altogether," says Maurer, "I have represented maybe forty or fifty clients over the course of time—some railway workers, some disability cases, some malpractice, and others involving forcing major medical [insurance] carriers to treat."

This last category is an important issue. Treatment with long-term intravenous antibiotics is an expensive proposition. Experts from the conventional side more often than not serve as consultants for the insurance industry, as it is in the industry's best interests not to pay for these expensive treatments. Some people in the alternative camp allege that doctors from the conventional camp and the industry are colluding to limit the benefits of subscribers ill with Lyme disease. The industry and the conventional camp respond that even of the patients who truly have Lyme disease, scientific evidence does not show that long-term antibiotics work.

"We do have some fundamental problems," Maurer acknowledges on this issue. "The fact of the matter is that the conservatives who adhere to the surveillance criteria to make a diagnosis and who work at major institutions control conferences and editorial boards. When these people point to the literature, it all supports their position."

As the 1990s drew to a close, legal issues heated up—and became more personal. The Massachusetts Board of Registration of Medicine received seven different complaints about Allen Steere in a fairly short period of time, a very large number for any one physician.

Looking at the dates on which the letters were received and considering their tone, one might conclude that they are the result of an orchestrated campaign to malign Steere's reputation. The complainants alleged that Steere misdiagnosed and improperly treated them. Ultimately, the board dismissed all seven complaints. However, the Massachusetts Lyme Disease Coalition, a community-based activist group, posted a letter on the Web dated March 1, 2000, that actively solicited complaints against Steere. The Web site says: "At present we have two substantial 'active' complaints. However it will take MANY MORE active complaints to trigger a full investigation and force the Board of Registration to open up their archives."

On the other side of the fence, Joseph Burrascano and others claim they have become the targets of an assault from the New York State Department of Health's Office of Professional Medical Conduct (OPMC). One doctor has already lost his license to practice medicine in New York because of Lyme disease–related controversy. Burrascano has referred to this process as "medical McCarthyism" and notes that the first he heard that he was being formally investigated was just two months after the Senate hearings in 1993 during which he openly stated his differences with the status quo. The OPMC notified him that he was being investigated after an anonymous complaint had been filed against him.

That was in 1994; the case against Burrascano remains open. At some of his hearings, many of his patients demonstrate their support of him and deny having given permission to the State of New York to confiscate their medical information.

The attacks on both Steere and Burrascano appear to be orchestrated assaults to decide medical policy in a political rather than a scientific arena. But the questions behind such discontent remain unanswered: Are some of the alternative camp doctors treating with too much antibiotics? What is the definition of "too much antibiotics"? Who decides this? In the end, it boils down to who defines the standard treatment. The alternative camp argues that the same small group of university-based physicians is trying to define this, pointing to research published in peer-reviewed literature; however, as Maurer pointed out, it is exactly these conventional camp physicians who are writing these articles and to some extent controlling their publication.

The February 6, 2002, issue of *JAMA* published an article titled "Relationships Between Authors of Clinical Practice Guidelines and the Pharmaceutical Industry." Clinical practice guidelines are written by groups of physicians, and these guidelines often are adopted or sponsored by large professional organizations. They are widely distributed and often form the basis for physicians' choices in drug therapy. The authors of this article surveyed nearly two hundred physicians who had written forty-four different practice guidelines for common diseases such as hypertension, heart attack, peptic ulcer, arthritis, and pneumonia. They chose these diseases for the reason that physicians writing practice guidelines for these particular diseases have the potential to affect tens or hundreds of thousands of other doctors and potentially influence their prescribing habits.

The researchers found that 87 percent of the authors of these clinical guidelines had some form of interaction with the pharmaceutical industry. More than half received financial support for their research, and more than a third of them had served as employees of or consultants to pharmaceutical companies. Nearly 60 percent worked with companies whose drugs were being considered in the clinical practice guideline. In 70 percent of the diseases they looked at, at least one author had a tie to drug companies.

Although it would be impossible for a survey to determine to what extent these relationships actually influenced the recommendations published in the guidelines, the researchers reported, "Seven percent thought that their own relationships with the pharmaceutical industry influenced their recommendations and 19 percent thought that their coauthors' recommendations were influenced by their relationships." Worse yet, "In published versions of the [guidelines], specific declarations regarding the personal financial interactions of individual authors with the pharmaceutical industry were made in only 2 cases [of 44]."

In addition to issues of who is on the committees that write treatment guidelines is the equally important issue of who is *not* represented. The Infectious Diseases Society of America is one group that publishes treatment guidelines on various diseases. These guidelines are published in major journals, are widely quoted in other journals, and greatly influence what physicians with average expertise prescribe. Dr. Sam Donta, an infectious diseases specialist and professor of medicine at Boston University School of Medicine, was initially on the committee for the practice guideline for Lyme disease. Philosophically aligned with the alternative camp, his views on the treatment of chronic Lyme disease were quite different from the views of the others on the committee, most of whom are aligned with the conventional camp. Because his viewpoint was not included in the final document, he removed his name from the list of authors. The final publication does not mention his work or his objections. It is as if the Supreme Court published only the majority opinion on a legal decision, and the dissenting opinion were not circulated and the dissenters were not identified.

How can these two differing sides communicate?

26 • An Independent Reality

In *The Structure of Scientific Revolutions,* Thomas Kuhn addresses the kind of jousting that occurs between two sides as paradigms collide: "When paradigms enter, as they must, into a debate about paradigm choice, their role is necessarily circular. Each group uses its own paradigm to argue in that paradigm's defense.

"The resulting circularity does not, of course, make the arguments wrong or even ineffectual. The man who premises a paradigm when arguing in its defense can nonetheless provide a clear exhibit of what scientific practice will be like for those who adopt the new view of nature. The exhibit can be immensely persuasive, often compellingly so. Yet, whatever its force, the status of the circular argument is only that of persuasion. It cannot be made logically or even probabilistically compelling for those who refuse to step into the circle."

This was best and most recently illustrated during the early days of the AIDS epidemic. Blood bank officials and CDC epidemiologists argued about applying the hepatitis B test to the U.S. blood supply because there was evidence that this would identify almost 90 percent of the blood infected with what we now call HIV, but at the time the virus had not been identified. The blood bank scientists repeatedly maintained that there was no proof that the blood supply was infected—there was no infectious agent, no direct test for the infectious agent, and no direct proof that the infected blood had caused AIDS.

Randy Shilts writes about this in his 1987 book *And the Band Played On:* "The blood industry continued to stonewall. A CDC study in the *New England Journal of Medicine* warned again of the problem of transfusion-related AIDS and was roundly criticized by blood bankers, who picked apart the methodology of the research." He continues, "in a January [1984] essay in the *New England Journal of Medicine,* industry spokesman Dr. Joseph Bove wrote, 'Whether the disease is caused by a transfusion-transmitted infectious agent is still unknown and will continue to be until further data are gathered and the agent isolated. . . . Patients should be reassured that blood banks are taking all possible steps to provide for safe blood transfusions.' "

Shilts documents that even when the CDC had counted seventy-three cases of transfusion-related AIDS, the blood bank industry would admit to only two of them and that "faithful medical writers almost unanimously followed the blood bankers' rhetoric that they were the first two adults diagnosed with transfusion AIDS in the United States."

To the epidemiologists, the evidence was crystal clear, albeit indirect and observational. These two groups argued from two different paradigms, and for quite some time they were unable to find sufficient common group on which to come to an agreement. This dispute was ultimately resolved both by advances in science (the virus was identified, tests were developed) and by public pressure.

At the century mark, still more information became available about Lyme disease; however, none of it closed the gap between opposing groups and their respective paradigms. In June 2001, the results of a study conducted under the auspices of the NIH were published in the *New England Journal of Medicine.* Dr. Mark Klempner, an infectious diseases specialist, was the principle investigator of this study aimed at determining whether long-term antibiotics helped patients with chronic Lyme disease. The study concluded that some patients who were treated for Lyme disease have persistent severe symptoms. The researchers, however, could find no evidence of persistent infection, by culture or by PCR. As well, they found that the percentage of patients who improved with antibiotics (about one-third) was the same as the percentage who improved while receiving a placebo.

These findings add wind to the sails of the conventional camp, who believe that long-term antibiotics are not indicated for patients with chronic Lyme disease who have already received what is considered to be an adequate course. And in fact, if one were to look at just the evidence that exists in the published medical literature, that evidence favors the conventional camp. But the findings did not end the debate between the groups, nor were they a death knell to the alternative paradigm. Says Dr. Sam Donta, who works at the same infectious diseases department at Boston University as Klempner, "they didn't show that other treatments wouldn't work. That [the specific doses of the specific antibiotics] is the same as other regimens is not proven. I would hope that people wouldn't conclude that one study should decide the whole field. It [their findings] begs the question on what's going on—psychosomatic, autoimmunity, lingering effects, or persistent infection?"

Donta raised further questions about the duration of antibiotics, the use of different antibiotics, and the use of additional drugs to make the antibiotics more effective. For instance, he believes that oral tetracycline is more effective than oral doxycycline. Although the two drugs are in the same family, they differ pharmacologically.

Enormous strides have been made over the past twenty-five years in defining, diagnosing, and understanding Lyme disease, but as of 2002, legitimate debate remains about the safety of the vaccine, the utility of long-term antibiotics, and the best way to diagnose the disease. Several studies are ongoing. Dr. Fallon, the psychiatrist who became interested in the psychiatric effects of Lyme disease, is pursuing another NIH-sponsored grant to study the effects of antibiotics on his patients.

Debate even persists about what Lyme disease is and is not. More than twenty-five years after what appeared to be a cluster of JRA in coastal Connecticut, disagreement still exists on this issue. Part of the CDC definition is physician-diagnosed EM; however, as discussed in Chapter 21, even though cases being diagnosed across the southern United States have physician-diagnosed EM, the CDC is calling this southern tick-associated rash illness rather than Lyme disease. Some have begun referring to the Lyme-like disease in the southern states as "Masters' disease," which both acknowledges Ed Masters's decade of work in this area and differentiates it from Lyme disease. Should Lyme disease be defined by the clinical marker of EM? Or should it be defined by the finding of a specific organism— *B. burgdorferi* sensu lato? If EM is no longer the crux of the definition, then the CDC surveillance criteria need to be changed. If it is associated only with a positive culture in the laboratory, then many cases of true Lyme disease would be discounted because cultures are sometimes negative and most physicians do not have access to them in any case.

Across the southern United States, the theme of biological diversity of borreliae has also become increasingly clear, although the advances have raised more questions than they have answered. There is the new borrelia that Barbour found in the Lone Star ticks, as well as other species, such as *B. andersoni* and *B. bisseti*. Almost certainly, many other species of *Borrelia* are yet to be identified, although not all will cause disease in humans.

In the borrelial disease relapsing fever, each tick species has its own borrelia associated with it. Each is a bit different biologically and has a different species name; furthermore, they may have different growth requirements in culture. Yet all of them cause the clinically defined disease that we call relapsing fever. Should this be the case also with Lyme disease?

The earth orbited the sun for untold millions of years before Copernicus and Galileo put forth that theory. Gravity exerted its force long before Newton proclaimed it so. Cholera killed thousands before Snow dismantled the Broad Street pump or Koch defined the comma-shaped bacillus. Women died from rampant streptococcal sepsis despite the status quo opinion that Semmelweis was wrong. Stomach ulcers were caused by *H. pylori* even while physicians suggested bland diets and doled out antacids and tranquilizers by the truckloads.

Both before and after the development and acceptance of the scientific method, practitioners of medicine and science have never been shy about advancing hypotheses. This is as it should be; generating hypotheses to test is fundamental to scientific advancement. Once a theory becomes the accepted truth, however, it becomes ingrained into the status quo. People will cling to it tenaciously and it is difficult to shake away, even in the face of new and compelling data.

Nature goes about its business quite independently of those humans who try to uncover its secrets. It does not reveal them easily. In fact, one can reasonably wonder about the meaning of "truth" when it comes to science and biology. Einstein's theory of relativity changed the prevailing vision of the truth that was constructed around Newtonian mechanics. What was true for Aristotle changed with Copernicus and Galileo, whose perceptions led to a quantum leap in our understanding of the truth. And even after that, Kepler made some minor revisions to the master Galileo's truth. This is the case for Lyme disease as for these other natural realities. The first children who came to their doctors with swollen inflamed knees were diagnosed with JRA. That was the paradigm in 1975; that was the best truth. Rashes were diagnosed as spider bites or cellulitis, again, conforming to the truth of the time.

It is always the work of individual people that advances our understanding of our complex and rich reality and leads to shifts in how we see our world. In the case of Lyme disease, many individuals have been tireless in their efforts. Polly Murray and Judith Mensch possessed the independence, tenacity, and perhaps instinct of a parent to question the truth as it existed in 1975. Lyme disease undoubtedly would have been recognized eventually without them, but their ability to question authority jump-started a process that might not have come for several more years. Mrs. Murray has continued to question authority and her resolve is still evident, as she remains active in the areas of Lyme disease education and discovery.

The two Navy doctors—William Burrows and William Mast— have not been directly involved with Lyme disease for some time. Burrows is chief dermatologist at the Scripps Clinic in La Jolla, San Diego, and Mast had an active gastroenterology practice in Chelmsford, Massachusetts, before recently retiring. Like Mrs. Murray and Mrs. Mensch, these men also were open-minded observers of their environment and possessed the curiosity to pursue something that others might have ignored.

Twenty-five years after meeting Polly Murray, Stephen Malawista remains a professor of medicine at Yale University and continues to research the disease that made his department one of the most productive Lyme disease research centers in the world. Many people who have gone on to other great discoveries began under Malawista's tutelage.

David Snydman moved to Tufts New England Medical Center in Boston shortly after his stint in public health in Connecticut. He practices infectious diseases there but does not specialize in Lyme disease.

Allen Steere moved from New Haven to Boston to become chief of his own rheumatology department. His lab has been responsible for many of the discoveries about Lyme disease, and he remains generally recognized as the world's foremost authority on the disease. At the same time, he remains the target of a smear campaign by some members of the alternative camp. He has resorted to hiring security guards for his public appearances and using special personnel to monitor threats made against his personal safety. In 2002, after fifteen years at Tufts University, he became head of rheumatology at the Massachusetts General Hospital, also in Boston.

Willy Burgdorfer continued his research into the organism that bears his name and, although officially retired, still works in his lab at the Rocky Mountain Laboratories and makes frequent appearances at the professional meetings on Lyme disease.

Andrew Spielman continues his work at the Harvard School of Public Health, and John Anderson still directs the Connecticut Agricultural Experiment Station. Both still research Lyme disease and other tick-borne diseases, as does Jorge Benach, who has remained an active researcher in this area.

Klaus Weber and Rudolph Ackermann, while both officially retired, also continue to work in the field and are preeminent European scientists in the Lyme disease field.

Ed Masters has continued his battle to have the Lyme-like disease in the South better recognized and better studied. Six years ago, critics claimed that he was simply misdiagnosing spider bites and making much ado about nothing. Although the precise language to describe what he has been observing for the past decade has yet to be elucidated, history has shown him to be a courageous observer and persistent scientist. Furthermore, at the Ninth International Conference on Lyme Borreliosis and Other Tick-Borne Diseases in New York City in August 2002, he was officially acknowledged.

Brian Fallon at Columbia continues his work exploring the psychiatric manifestations of Lyme disease.

Joseph Burrascano Jr. is still embroiled in his legal battle but remains a popular doctor for numerous patients who feel that they have not received the right answers from more conventional doctors.

Karen Forschner and her husband Tom continue to advance their cause in the political arena.

On February 25, 2002, GlaxoSmithKline discontinued selling LYMErix, not because it was potentially unsafe but because the company considered sales to be "insufficient to justify the continued investment in manufacturing, distribution and marketing."

An enormous amount of investigative work has taken place during the past century regarding Lyme disease. Much of the work done over the past twenty-five years has been brilliant and some of it inspired. Doctors and scientists of all stripes have peeled away many of nature's secrets, but not all of them. The notion that we fully understand Lyme disease as of the year 2002 is at best wishful thinking; at worst, it illustrates a hubris that is uniquely human. In the early 1970s, for instance, complacency about infectious diseases developed. We believed we had powerful antibiotics that could kill any bug, and some people went so far as to think that we had won the battle against infectious agents.

Nothing could be further from the truth. Just during the past quarter century, in addition to Lyme disease, babesiosis, and ehrlichiosis, we have seen AIDS, Legionnaire's disease, toxic shock syndrome, Hantavirus, new *E. coli* infections of the intestine, Ebola virus, Lassa fever, West Nile encephalitis, and other new infectious diseases. In addition to these emerging diseases, ancient killers such as malaria, tuberculosis, and African sleeping sickness infect and take the lives of millions of children and adults every year. Hepatitis C is another modern epidemic with disastrous consequences. Cholera still kills. Dengue fever is on the upswing throughout the Caribbean and the Americas. After September 11, 2001, anthrax, a disease that we thought to be exceedingly rare, and smallpox, thought to be eradicated decades ago, are once again perceived as real threats. And there will be new microbial adversaries that we have not yet discovered and for which we do not yet have names.

In short, our understanding of Lyme disease is by definition limited. Remember Joe Dowhan, the first patient who brought in the *I. scapularis* tick, who began experiencing neurological symptoms thirteen years after his initial infection. Where was the spirochete all of this time? Malawista is still working on this problem, likening long periods of time when a patient has no symptoms to "Sherlock Holmes' dog that did not bark. What is the immune system if not a guard dog? Why has it stopped responding to the spirochetes in its midst?"

Such limitations to our knowledge could change next week, next year, next decade, or they might require another twenty-five years of work. More likely, our understanding will undergo numerous revisions over time. And there will be other curious people who notice strange goings-on, other patients with baffling arrays of symptoms that do not seem to match known patterns. Unraveling the continuing mysteries of Lyme disease and solving the new puzzles that nature throws our way will require a commitment to uncovering and then analyzing new data as they arise.

Our collective approach, as a society, to newly recognized disease threats is an important part of our public health system. How we respond to these threats will largely determine how quickly we protect ourselves from them. We must strive to minimize the politics of these battles and maximize the science. We must strive to keep the science as ethically clean as possible. Perhaps the most dangerous thing of all, to our patients, to ourselves, and to science, is to pretend to know what we really do not.

• Epilogue

As this book went to press, I attended the Ninth International Conference on Lyme Borreliosis and Other Tick-Borne Diseases during August 2002. The conference had evolved considerably from the first one in New Haven in 1983. Five hundred participants (approximately three to four times the original number) from more than thirty-one states and thirty countries (up from thirteen states and four countries in 1983) came to New York to share ideas and present data. Many of the names with which the reader is now familiar were present—Drs. Steere, Malawista, Barbour, Benach, Ackermann, Masters, Fallon, and others.

The participants shared information about a wealth of scientific advances that had occurred since the last international conference in Munich in 1999. Genetic analysis has showed that even more individual species of *B. burgdorferi* exist than had been previously realized, although it is not clear that all of them cause disease in humans. Scientists have increasingly learned more about the biology of the spirochete, but to date, *B. burgdorferi* continues to keep many of its secrets. The genetic diversity of borreliae was apparent, and some, including Malawista, suggested ways that this biological diversity might play a role in the cause of Lyme arthritis.

One presenter wondered whether Koch's postulates require revision in this age of genetic sequencing of entire genomes and PCR diagnosis by amplifying the tiniest strands of DNA. Causality in medicine has descended to the molecular and submolecular level.

Regarding diagnostic testing, new antigens, named C6 and Vlse, that appear to be quite specific for *B. burgdorferi* show great promise. Although not quite ready for prime time, serologic tests made from these antigens seem to be both simpler and possibly more accurate than the current CDC-recommended two-step system of ELISA and Western blot. They may help with diagnosis in Europe as well. European researchers presented data that showed a greater biodiversity in their borreliae, complicating their search for an ideal diagnostic test as well as for a vaccine. Some presenters discussed why the vaccine failed and what lessons have been learned from that experience.

As the title of the conference indicates, more emphasis was placed on coinfections with other tick-borne pathogens, especially babesiosis and ehrlichiosis. Since the sections in this book were written that deal with ehrlichiosis, taxonomists have changed the scientific name of the agent of human granulocytic ehrlichiosis from *E. equi* to *Anaplasma phagocytophila*. The increasing use of genetics and DNA and RNA analysis is changing the way that scientists group organisms.

There was a great deal of discussion about Masters' disease, and at one point, all five hundred attendees recognized Ed Masters's role and persistence by giving him a round of applause—a poignant moment for a man who less than a decade ago was being ridiculed for his beliefs by some of the people in that assembly.

Many presentations were concerned with treatment, and within the conference, there was a clear trend toward shorter rather than longer lengths of antibiotic therapy. The large majority of participants approved when Mark Klempner presented his study (see Chapter 26) about the lack of effect of long-term antibiotics.

At the same time, there were some difficult realities. Security was orders of magnitude tighter than for any other of the dozens of medical conferences I have attended over two decades. Outside of the conference, I learned why. Across the street, approximately 150 demonstrators from the alternative camp stood behind a police barricade, holding signs and distributing pamphlets that challenged the scientific evidence being presented inside.

Even within the conference, a few tense moments arose. Moderators did not give the floor to physicians aligned with the alternative camp who tried to make comments, even though their conventional camp colleagues had been afforded that courtesy. At one point, when a physician aligned with the alternative camp, whose comments were about to be cut short, suggested that the purpose of a scientific meeting was to discuss differences of opinion, another participant shouted out that information was being suppressed. So although discussion, conversation, and some sharing of views occurred, clear signs of persisting animosity between the groups remained.

This conference took place nearly 120 years after Alfred Buchwald's description of ACA, more than ninety years after Arvid Afzelius's initial description of EM, and more than twenty-five years after the statistically improbable cluster of what was thought to be JRA by doctors in coastal Connecticut. We still have a lot to learn about Lyme disease, and more importantly, we still have a lot to learn about the scientific process.

SYMPTOMS OF LYME DISEASE

This lists common symptoms seen during the acute and later stages of the disease. It is not meant to be encyclopedic.

Early localized disease (usually occur days to weeks after tick bite)
- Erythema migrans (a large red rash)
- Fever and chills
- Headache and neck stiffness

Early disseminated disease (usually occur weeks to months after tick bite)
- Multiple erythema migrans lesions
- Borrelial lymphocytoma (nearly exclusively in Europe)
- Neurological
  —Bell's palsy
  —Radiculoneuritis (inflammation of nerve roots as they exit the spinal cord)
  —Aseptic meningitis
- Cardiac involvement (palpitations, slow heart beat)
- Arthritis (joint swelling and pain; far more common in late disease)

Late disease (usually occur months to years after tick bite)
- Arthritis
- Rash (acrodermatitis chronicum atrophicans; nearly exclusively in Europe)
- Neurological syndromes
  —Neuropathy (pains and abnormal sensations, sometimes with weakness in the extremities)
  —Encephalopathy (problems with memory; altered mood, sleep, and cognitive functions)

TICK-BORNE DISEASES IN HUMANS AND ANIMALS

Disease	Host	Tick Vector	Agent
Lyme disease	Humans, animals	*Ixodes* ticks (various species)	*Borrelia burgdorferi* *B. afzelii* *B. garinii* Unknown others in the southern United States
Masters' disease (also called southern tick-associated rash illness or STARI)	Humans	*Amblyomma americanum*	Unknown, likely a novel *Borrelia*
Babesiosis	Humans, animals	*Ixodes* ticks (various species)	*Babesia microti* (humans in North America) *B. divergens* (humans in Europe) *B. gibsoni* (dogs)
Human granulocytic and monocytic ehrlichiosis	Humans	*Ixodes* ticks *Amblyomma* ticks	*E. equi, ewingii* *E. chafeensis*
Rocky Mountain spotted fever	Humans	*Dermacentor* ticks	*Rickettsia rickettsiae*
Mediterranean (boutonneuse fever) and other spotted fevers	Humans	*Rhipicephalus* ticks (in Europe)	*Rickettsia connorii* (and others)
Colorado tick fever	Humans	*Dermacentor andersoni*	Colorado tick fever virus (an RNA coltivirus)
Relapsing fever	Humans	*Ornithodoros* ticks (various species)	*Borrelia* (various species, each specific to a particular tick species)
Tularemia	Humans, animals	*Dermacentor* and *Amblyomma* ticks	*Francisella tularensis*
Q fever	Humans, animals	Various	*Coxiella burnetii*
Tick-borne encephalitis	Humans (Europe)	*Ixodes ricinus* *I. persulcatus*	Central European encephalitis virus (CEE)

Disease	Host	Tick Vector	Agent
Tick-borne (Powassan) encephalitis	Humans (North America)	*Ixodes scapularis*	Powassan virus (analogue of CEE)
Tick paralysis	Humans	Various (depends on region)	Toxin
Texas cattle fever	Cattle	*Dermacentor*	*Babesia* species
Bovine anaplasmosis	Cattle		*Ehrlichia* species
Heartwater fever, or cowdriosis	Cattle		*Ehrlichia* species
Canine ehrlichiosis	Dogs		*Ehrlichia* species

Note: Only the animal tick-borne diseases mentioned in the text are included. Diseases that can occur in both humans and animals are listed once and so noted in the Host column.

For brevity and simplicity, when multiple authors contributed to a source, only the name of the first author is included.

CHAPTER 1 • A FAMILY UNDER SIEGE

I interviewed Polly Murray on at least three occasions, both by telephone and in her home in Connecticut, during 1988, 1993, and 2001. She and I had the opportunity of speaking on several other occasions as well. I also have quoted directly both from her book *The Widening Circle* (New York: St. Martins Press, 1996) and from a letter she wrote to the editor of the *New England Journal of Medicine* (vol. 305 [1981]: 895). I also spoke with her son, Todd Murray, by telephone in 2001. In addition, I interviewed Dr. Peter Schur, a rheumatologist at the Brigham and Woman's Hospital in Boston in 1994.

CHAPTER 2 • A LITTLE GIRL'S KNEE

I interviewed Judith Mensch by telephone twice in 1993 and also found useful information in an article titled "Lyme disease" that she wrote and published in the *Maryland Medical Journal* in 1985 (vol. 34: 691–92), in which she describes some of her role in the discovery of Lyme disease. I spoke by telephone with Aileen Paterson in 1994 and again in 2001. For some of the information relating to rheumatic fever and juvenile rheumatoid arthritis, I used standard textbooks of rheumatology and internal medicine as well as *Pediatric Emergency Medicine,* a standard emergency medicine textbook edited by Roger Barkin (St. Louis: Mosby, 1992). I also quote from Sir William Osler's *Principles and Practice of Medicine* (1st ed., New York: D. Appleton and Co., 1899).

CHAPTER 3 • THE BROAD STREET PUMP

The details of John Snow's investigation of cholera are from a reprint of his work called *Snow on Cholera—Being a Reprint of Two Papers,* edited by William Frost (New York: The Commonwealth Fund, 1936). This is a fascinating epidemiological tale to read. Two other books rounded out the facts on cholera: *Some Notable Epidemics,* written by Harold Scott (London: Edward Arnold & Co., 1934), and Charles-Edward Winslow's *The Conquest of Epidemic Disease* (Madison: University of Wisconsin Press, 1980). I found information about the CDC's Epidemiology Intelligence Service in an issue of *JAMA* in 2001 (vol. 285: 1947–49). I also got a sense of this from interviews with former EIS agent Dr. John Hanrahan of Boston. As well, I interviewed Dr. David Snydman in both 1994 and 2001 in his office in Boston. He kindly allowed me access to his original written notes, reports, and case finding map that he used to track the fledgling epidemic.

CHAPTER 4 · AN APPOINTMENT IN NEW HAVEN

The information attributed to Polly Murray is from the above-mentioned interviews and from her book (Chapter 1). I communicated with Dr. Stephen Malawista in 1994 in New Haven, and again in 2002, both by E-mail and in New York City. I also interviewed Dr. Allen Steere twice in his office at New England Medical Center in Boston in 1994.

CHAPTER 5 · AN OUTBREAK OF ARTHRITIS

Some of the quotations come from the aforementioned interviews with Drs. Steere and Malawista. I also quote from the original article describing Lyme arthritis, "Lyme arthritis: an epidemic of oligoarticular arthritis in children and adults in three Connecticut communities," which was published in *Arthritis and Rheumatism* in 1977 (vol. 20: 7–17). I spoke by telephone with two other authors of that manuscript— Dr. Warren Andiman from Yale University and Dr. Robert Shope, currently at the University of Texas at Galveston. Some of the background information on tropical diseases comes from the wonderful review of tropical diseases by Dr. Mary Wilson, *A World Guide to Infections* (New York: Oxford University Press, 1991).

CHAPTER 6 · AN OUTBREAK OF DERMATITIS

I interviewed Drs. William Mast and William Burrows individually by telephone in 1994. I also used their original publication of cases of erythema migrans that was published in *JAMA* in 1976 ("Erythema chronicum migrans in the United States," vol. 236: 859–60). I spoke with several dermatologists who played a role in the story. One was Dr. Thomas Hansen, who was in private practice when I spoke with him in 1994. That same year, I also spoke with Dr. Irwin Braverman, who headed Yale's Dermatology Division in the mid-1970s. Last, I talked with Dr. Rudolph Scrimenti, from Milwaukee, by telephone in 1994 and in person in 1997. He described the first case of EM in an article in the *Archives of Dermatology* in 1970 ("Erythema chronicum migrans," vol. 102: 104–5). Scrimenti also wrote an article called "Lyme disease redux: the legacy of Sven Hellerstrom" published in the *Wisconsin Medical Journal* (vol. 92 [1993]: 20–21). I read Hellerstrom's original paper titled "Erythema chronicum migrans Afzelius with meningitis," which was published in the *Southern Medical Journal* (vol. 43 [1950]: 330–35). In 1994, I spoke by telephone with Dr. Edgar Grunwaldt, a physician on Shelter Island, New York, who found himself unexpectedly in the middle of an epidemic.

CHAPTER 7 • THE EUROPEAN CONNECTION

The work in Europe is an important and less well-known part of the story of Lyme disease. I found the single best source of this history in the chapter called "History of Lyme Borreliosis in Europe," written by Drs. Klaus Weber and Hans-Walter Pfister in the book *Aspects of Lyme Borreliosis,* edited by Weber and Willy Burgdorfer (Berlin: Springer-Verlag, 1992). I communicated with Weber on several occasions, once in Munich in 1999 and again in 2002, both electronically and by telephone. I also reviewed Arvid Afzelius's landmark contribution titled "Verhandlungen der Dermatologischen Gesellshaft zu Stockholm," which was published in 1910 in the *Archives of Dermatology and Syphilis* (vol. 101: 404). Harvard pathologist Gustav Dammin wrote a nice article, "Erythema migrans: a chronicle," that was published in the *Review of Infectious Diseases* in 1989 (vol. 11: 142–51). The original report by Dr. Charles Garin and A. Bujadoux titled "Paralysis by ticks" that was published in the *Medical Journal of Lyon* was reprinted in *Clinical Infectious Diseases* in 1993 (vol. 16: 168–69).

CHAPTER 8 • FURTHER WORK IN EUROPE

In addition to Weber and Pfister's chapter mentioned above (Chapter 7), I reviewed several other articles and books to gather further information on research on the European side of the Atlantic. Carl Lennhoff published his work with spirochetes as the etiology of obscure diseases in *Acta Dermatologica & Venereology* (Stockholm) in 1948 (vol. 28: 295–324). It is a long article but one that has many interesting details. Nils Thyresson also shares some interesting details in his article "Historical notes on skin manifestations of Lyme borreliosis," published in 1991 in the *Scandinavian Journal of Infectious Diseases* (vol. 77 [suppl]: 9–13). Another original article that served as a noteworthy source for this chapter is by Dr. Alfred Buchwald, the German physician who was the very first to report on any manifestation of what is now known to be Lyme disease—the skin rash ACA. He published this case report called "Ein Fall von diffuser idiopathischer Haut-Atrophie" in 1883 in the *Archives of Dermatology & Syphilis* (Wien) (vol. 10: 553–56).

I referred to three books for this chapter. The first is *Biography of a Germ,* by Arno Karlen (New York: Pantheon Books, 2000)—a fascinating book about *B. burgdorferi* as seen from the perspective of the spirochete. The data on the discovery of penicillin derive from another informative book, *Medicine's Ten Greatest Discoveries,* by Meyer Friedman and Gerald Friedland (New Haven: Yale University Press, 1968). The last book, *Who Goes First?,* devotes itself to the history of self-experimentation by physicians and is written by Lawrence Altman (New York: Random House, 1986).

CHAPTER 9 • THE BLIND MEN AND THE ELEPHANT

Chapter 9 makes use of some of the first articles by Allen Steere and colleagues, including the one mentioned in Chapter 5. Their next major article, "Erythema chronicum migrans and Lyme arthritis: the enlarging clinical spectrum," was published in the *Annals of Internal Medicine* in 1977 (vol. 86: 685–98). I also used the interviews of Steere, Malawista, Mast, and Burrows mentioned above, as well as the report in *JAMA* by the latter two (Chapter 6).

Articles from lay newspapers helped to fill in some of the details of the time—specifically, Boyce Rensberger in the *New York Times* (July 18, 1976), David Heckerman's report in the *New London Day* (July 28, 1976), and Kyn Tolson's piece from the *Old Lyme Gazette* (July 29, 1976) and another piece in *The Star* (June 1976). I also quote from a letter dated May 18, 1976, sent by Steere and Malawista to the patients who participated in the study (graciously supplied to me by Polly Murray). Mrs. Murray also spoke with me about these incidents.

CHAPTER 10 • THE CONNECTION WITH TICKS

I interviewed Joe Dowhan by telephone in 1994, and he supplied some spectacular details concerning his tick bites more than twenty years earlier. The background on ticks comes from a 1965 article by D. Arthur in *Nature* called "Ticks in Egypt in 1500 B.C.?" (vol. 206: 1060–61). Other details come from Berton Roueche's *New Yorker* piece from 1988 titled "The foulest and nastiest creatures that be" (September 12, pages 83–89). Much of the ecological data in this and later chapters is from the chapter called "The origins and course of the present outbreak of Lyme disease," written by Andrew Spielman and colleagues in the book *Ecology and Environmental Management of Lyme Disease,* edited by Howard Ginsberg (New Brunswick, N.J.: Rutgers University Press, 1993). Hans Zinsser's book *Rats, Lice and History* (New York: Black Dog and Leventhal, 1934) is an erudite study of typhus fever and excellent reading for students of the history of medicine.

CHAPTER 11 • AN INTERSECTION OF INVESTIGATIONS

I interviewed Jorge Benach (by telephone, 1994, and personally in New York, 2002), John Anderson (New Haven, 2001), Willy Burgdorfer (on several occasions by telephone and in person in New York, Vancouver, and Munich), Steve Dumler (1998), Andrew Spielman (1993 in Boston), and Edgar Grunwaldt (by telephone, 1994). I read Anderson's article "The natural history of ticks" in *Medical Clinics of North America* on the natural history of ticks (Saunders, vol. 86 [2002]: 205–18); R. Wallis's field study of ticks and Lyme arthritis, "Erythema chronicum migrans and Lyme arthritis: field study of ticks" in the *American Journal of Epidemiology* (vol. 108 [1978]: 322–27); Steere's article on the early epidemiology of Lyme disease, "Erythema chronicum migrans and Lyme arthritis: epidemiologic evidence for a tick vector," also published in the *American Journal of Epidemiology* (vol. 108 [1978]: 312–27); K. Western's article about the index case of babesiosis on Nantucket Island, "Babesiosis in a Massachusetts resident," published in the *New England Journal of Medicine* (vol. 283 [1970]: 854–56); and Anderson's "Canine babesia new to North America" from *Science* (vol. 204 [1979]: 1431–32).

Some of the articles on Rocky Mountain spotted fever included J. S. Dumler's "Fatal Rocky Mountain spotted fever in Maryland—1901," published in *JAMA* (vol. 265 [1991]: 718); Gerald Hazard's "Rocky Mountain spotted fever in the eastern United States" in the *New England Journal of Medicine* (vol. 280 [1969]: 57–62); Benach's "Changing patterns in the incidence of Rocky Mountain spotted fever on Long Island (1971–1976)" in the *American Journal of Epidemiology* (vol. 106 [1977]: 380–87); Burgdorfer's "A review of Rocky Mountain spotted fever, its agent and its tick vectors in the United States," published in the *Journal of Medical Entomology* (vol. 12 [1975]: 269–78); and Louis Magnarelli's "Rocky Mountain spotted fever in Connecticut: human cases, spotted fever group rickettsiae in ticks, and antibodies in mammals," in the *American Journal of Epidemiology* (vol. 110 [1979]: 148–55). Edgar Grunwaldt's article "Babesiosis on Shelter Island," published in 1977 in the *New York State Journal of Medicine* (vol. 77: 1320–21), is rather interesting given the early date of publication.

Victoria Harden's book *Rocky Mountain Spotted Fever: History of a Twentieth Century Disease* (Baltimore: Johns Hopkins University Press, 1990) provided much interesting history of rickettsial diseases and the people who study them. I recommend it for anyone interested in the history of medicine.

CHAPTER 12 • FROM THE ALPS TO THE ROCKIES

Willy Burgdorfer wrote many of the articles that I used for primary source material, and some of the blanks were filled in by the aforementioned interviews and telephone calls with him. His articles include the following: "How the discovery of *B. burgdorferi* came about" (*Clinics in Dermatology*, Saunders, vol. 11 [1993]: 335–38); "The historical road to the discovery of *B. burgdorferi*" in the book *Aspects of Lyme Borreliosis*, edited by Burgdorfer and Weber (Berlin: Springer-Verlag, 1992); and "Discovery of the Lyme disease spirochete: a historical review" (*Zentralblatt Bakteriologie, Mikrobiologie & Hygiene [A]*, vol. 262 [1986]: 7–10). Burgdorfer also had a speech of his published in the *Review of Infectious Diseases* (vol. 8 [1986]: 932–39) called "The enlarging spectrum of tick-borne spirochetoses: R. R. Parker memorial address."

Background on the outbreak of relapsing fever in Washington was found in the report "Outbreak of tick-borne relapsing fever in Spokane County, Washington," by R. Thompson, who published the events in *JAMA* (vol. 210 [1969]: 1045–50). As regards the history of the biology of borreliae, I heavily used Alan Barbour's "Cultivation of Borrelia: a historical review," written in 1986 and published in *Zentralblatt Bakteriologie, Mikrobiologie & Hygiene [A]* (vol. 263: 11–14), and Richard Kelly's "Cultivation of Borrelia hermsii," published in 1971 in *Science* (vol. 173: 443–44).

The background on Robert Koch comes both from the Nobel Prize Web site (http://www.nobel.se) and from Charles-Edward Winslow's book *The Conquest of Epidemic Disease* (Madison: University of Wisconsin Press, 1980).

CHAPTER 13 • TO TREAT OR NOT TO TREAT?

I used a series of articles first authored by Barry Marshall regarding his work on the etiology of peptic ulcers: "Attempt to fulfill Koch's postulates for pyloric *Campylobacter*" (*Medical Journal of Australia*, vol. 142 [1985]: 436–39), "The Campylobacter pylori story" (*Scandinavian Journal of Gastroenterology*, vol. 146 [suppl, 1988]: 58–66), "Helicobacter pylori: the etiologic agent for peptic ulcer" (*JAMA*, vol. 274 [1995]: 1064–66), "Helicobacter pylori in peptic ulcer: have Koch's postulates been fulfilled?" (*Annals of Medicine*, vol. 27 [1995]: 565–68), "The future of Helicobacter pylori eradication: a personal perspective" (*Alimentary Pharmacology and Therapy*, vol. 11 [suppl, 1997]: 109–15), and "Helicobacter pylori: 20 years on" (*Clinical Medicine*, vol. 2 [2002]: 147–52. Collectively, these articles make great reading for anyone who possesses an interest in scientific discovery.

I also used Spielman's article "Human babesiosis on Nantucket Island, USA: description of the vector, *Ixodes dammini*, n. sp. (acarina: Ixodidae)" in the *Journal of Medical Entomology* (vol. 15 [1979]: 218–34). The information about Grunwaldt comes both from my interview of him and from quoted material from the aforementioned Roueche article in the *New Yorker* (Chapter 10). The Yale group's article published in 1980 in the *Annals of Internal Medicine* titled "Antibiotic therapy in Lyme disease" (vol. 93: 1–8) rounded out some of the issues on therapy, as did the interviews of Steere and Malawista mentioned above. I also spoke with Dr. Richard Root by telephone in 2001; he was the chief of infectious diseases at Yale during the mid-1970s.

CHAPTER 14 • THE SCRAMBLE FOR THE CAUSE

I interviewed both Dr. George Schmid by telephone and Dr. John Hanrahan in Boston in 2001 and also used information from the aforementioned interviews of Steere and Anderson. Schmid authored an article about the newly recognized leptospire published in 1986 in the *Clinical Journal of Microbiology* (vol. 24: 484–86).

I begin to discuss serologic testing in this chapter, and the information comes from many sources. I especially direct the lay reader to Alan Barbour's book *Lyme Disease: The Cause, the Cure, the Controversy* (Baltimore: Johns Hopkins University Press, 1996). Three more technical accounts are by Louis Magnarelli ("Current status of laboratory diagnosis of Lyme disease," *American Journal of Medicine*, vol. 98 [suppl, 1995]: 10S–14S), the American College of Physicians ("Guide for laboratory evaluation in the diagnosis of Lyme disease," *Annals of Internal Medicine*, vol. 127 [1997]: 1106–8), and Johan Bunikis and Alan Barbour ("Laboratory testing for suspected Lyme disease," *Medical Clinics of North America*, Saunders, vol. 86 [2002]:

311–40). The European perspective comes from 2001 interviews with and letters by Klaus Weber and Rudolph Ackermann. As well, Weber's 1974 article titled "ECM meningitis—a bacterial infectious disease?" from the *Münchener Medizinische Wochenschrift* (vol. 116: 1993–98) and his 1981 article in *Dermatology* ("Serological study with rickettsial antigens in erythema chronicum migrans," vol. 163: 460–67) describe much of the etiologic considerations in this chapter. I also used his chapter mentioned above in the book that he and Burgdorfer edited (*Aspects of Lyme Borreliosis*, Chapter 7).

CHAPTER 15 • THE CULMINATION OF EFFORTS

· For the story about finding the spirochete, I refer the reader to an exceptional magazine article written by Joel Lang called "Catching the bug: how scientists found the cause of Lyme disease and why we're not out of the woods yet." It was reprinted in *Connecticut Medicine* in 1989 (vol. 53: 357–64) and is very much worth reading. I relied on the previously referenced interviews of Benach, Barbour, Burgdorfer, Grunwaldt, Hanrahan, Weber, and Ackermann.

The three prime articles on etiology in the United States that I used were Burgdorfer's "Lyme disease—a tick-borne spirochetosis?" from *Science* (vol. 216 [1983]: 1317–19), Steere's "The spirochetal etiology of Lyme disease" from the *New England Journal of Medicine* (vol. 308 [1983]: 733–40), and Benach's "Spirochetes isolated from the blood of two patients with Lyme disease," also from the *New England Journal of Medicine* (vol. 308 [1983]: 740–42). John Anderson and colleagues also published at about the same time the article "Spirochetes in *Ixodes dammini* and mammals from Connecticut" in the *American Journal of Tropical Medicine and Hygiene* (vol. 32 [1983]: 818–24).

On the European side of the equation, Ackermann published four articles about his findings on ECM and the new spirochete: "Chronic erythema migrans and tick-transmitted meningopolyneuritis (Garin-Bujadoux-Bannwarth): Borrelia infections?" (in German) (*Deutsche Medizinische Wochenschraft*, vol. 108 [1983]: 577–79), "Spirochete etiology of erythema chronicum migrans disease" (in German) (*Deutsche Medizinische Wochenschraft*, vol. 109 [1984]: 92–97), "The spirochetal etiology of erythema chronicum migrans and of meningo-polyneuritis Garin-Bujadoux-Bannwarth" (in German) (*Zeitschrift fur Hautkrankheiten*), vol. 58 [1983]: 1619–21), and "*Ixodes ricinus* spirochete and European erythema chronicum migrans disease" (*Yale Journal of Biology and Medicine*, vol. 57 [1984]: 573–80). I read A. Stewart's article on Lyme disease in Australia published in 1982 in the *Medical Journal of Australia* ("Lyme arthritis in the Hunter Valley," vol. 1: 139).

CHAPTER 16 • PROGRESS TO THE END OF THE 1980s

This chapter contains information detailed in the transcripts of the First International Symposium on Lyme Disease held in New Haven in 1983 and published by the *Yale Journal of Biology and Medicine* (vol. 57 [1984]: 445–713). Some of this information is the perspective of Polly Murray in her aforementioned book *The Widening Circle*. Interviews of Barbour, Burgdorfer, Anderson, Weber, Dr. Russell Johnson, and Dr. James Oliver also provided much-needed perspective on events around the conference.

I spoke briefly with Dr. David Persing about his role in using PCR analysis for diagnostic testing and read his article "Polymerase chain reaction: trenches to benches" published in the *Journal of Clinical Microbiology* in 1991 (vol. 29: 1281–85). A book that I used to better understand PCR and one that I highly recommend to the scientifically oriented and lay reader alike is the highly informative and entertaining *Dancing Naked in the Mind Field* (New York: Vantage Books, 1998), by Dr. Kary Mullis, the inventor of PCR. Five articles detail the results of the PCR search to determine the antiquity of the borrelia that causes Lyme disease. Two were authored by Persing: "Detection of *Borrelia burgdorferi* in *Ixodes dammini* ticks with the PCR" (*Journal of Clinical Microbiology*, vol. 28 [1990]: 566–72) and "Detection of *Borrelia burgdorferi* DNA in museum specimens of *Ixodes dammini* ticks" (*Science*, vol. 249 [1990]: 1420–23). Franz-Rainer Matuschka wrote two: "Characteristics of Lyme disease spirochetes in archived European ticks" (*Journal of Infectious Diseases*, vol. 174 [1996]: 424–26) and "Antiquity of the Lyme disease spirochete in Europe" (*Lancet*, vol. 346 [1995]: 1367). The fifth is by Jerzy Tobolewski, "Detection and identification of mammalian DNA from the gut of museum specimens of ticks" (*Journal of Medical Entomology*, vol. 29 [1992]: 1049–51).

The two major articles on the naming of the tick (deer tick versus black-legged tick or *Ixodes dammini* versus *Ixodes scapularis*) are the aforementioned Spielman article "Human babesiosis on Nantucket Island, USA" (Chapter 13) and one by James Oliver, "Conspecificity of the ticks Ixodes scapularis and I. dammini (Acari: Ixodidae), in the *Journal of Medical Entomology* (vol. 30 [1993]: 54–63).

CHAPTER 17 • A GEOGRAPHICAL EXPANSION

Many of the ecological details come from Spielman's chapter in the Ginsberg book mentioned above (Chapter 10). Some of the information about the history of forest cover comes from the Ohio Department of Natural Resources Web site at http://www.dnr.state.oh.us/forestry/forest/ohiogreen.htm. Much of the data on incidence comes from tallies kept on the CDC's Web site http://www.cdc.gov.

I used epidemiological data from the following articles: "Physician reporting of Lyme disease—Connecticut, 1991–92" (*Morbidity and Mortality Weekly Reports*, vol. 42: 348–57), B. S. Coyle's "The public health impact of Lyme disease in Maryland" (*Journal of Infectious Diseases*, vol. 173 [1996]: 1260–62), Steere's "Cases of Lyme disease in the United States: locations correlated with distribution of *Ixodes dammini*"

(*Annals of Internal Medicine,* vol. 91 [1979]: 730–33), George Schmid's "Surveillance of Lyme disease in the United States" (*Journal of Infectious Diseases,* vol. 151 [1985]: 1144–49), Catherine Lastavica's "Rapid emergence of a focal epidemic of Lyme disease in coastal Massachusetts" (*New England Journal of Medicine,* vol. 320 [1989]: 133–37), Dennis White's interesting article on the spread in New York state called "The geographic spread and temporal increase of the Lyme disease epidemic" (*JAMA,* vol. 266 [1991]: 1230–36), and Robert Smith's "Role of bird migration in the long-distance dispersal of *Ixodes dammini,* the vector of Lyme disease" (*Journal of Infectious Diseases,* vol. 174 [1996]: 221–24). I also interviewed James Oliver (2001, by telephone) and Ed Masters (telephone, 1994) and read the article by Masters, "Erythema migrans—rash as key to early diagnosis of Lyme disease," from *Postgraduate Medicine* (vol. 94 [1993]: 133–34, 137–42).

CHAPTER 18 • THE DIAGNOSTICIAN'S DILEMMA

Most of the information comes from standard statistics and is generally known. Two particular articles cover some of this information as it specifically relates to Lyme disease: Phil Tugwell's "Laboratory evaluation in the diagnosis of Lyme disease" (*Annals of Internal Medicine,* vol. 127 [1997]: 1109–23) and G. Nichol's "Test-treatment strategies for patients suspected of having Lyme disease: a cost-effectiveness analysis" (*Annals of Internal Medicine,* vol. 128 [1998]: 37–48).

CHAPTER 19 • AMBIGUITY IN THE LAB

Alan Barbour's book (mentioned above, Chapter 14) has an excellent treatment of laboratory diagnosis, as does the article he co-wrote with Bunikis (also above, Chapter 14). The theme of laboratory variation is covered by L. Bakken's "Performance of 45 laboratories participating in a proficiency testing program for Lyme disease serology" published in *JAMA* (vol. 268 [1992]: 891–95) and Steve Luger's "Serologic tests for Lyme disease: interlaboratory variability," published in the *Archives of Internal Medicine* (vol. 150 [1990]: 761–63). Steere covers the same issues in his *New England Journal Review* article "Lyme disease" (vol. 345 [2001]: 115–25). In 1995, the CDC published its recommendations of the two-step testing strategy, "Recommendations for test performance and interpretation from the Second National Conference on serologic diagnosis of Lyme disease," in *Morbidity and Mortality Weekly Review* (vol. 44: 590–91). Dr. Paul Fawcett also helped me understand some of the intricacies of these tests during a telephone interview conducted in 2001.

CHAPTER 20 • A TICK WITH TWO TOXINS

Numerous articles published on various tick-borne pathogens were helpful and are listed here: Paul Mitchell's "Immunoserologic evidence of coinfection with *Borrelia burgdorferi, Babesia microti,* and human granulocytic Ehrlichia species in residents of Wisconsin and Minnesota" (*Journal of Clinical Microbiology,* vol. 34 [1996]: 724–27), Juan Olano's "Human ehrlichiosis" (*Medical Clinics of North America,* vol. 86 [2002]: 375–92), Peter Krause's "Concurrent Lyme disease and babesiosis: evidence for increased severity and duration of illness" (*JAMA,* vol. 275 [1996]: 1657–60), T. Wang's "Coexposure to *Borrelia burgdorferi* and *Babesis microti* does not worsen the long-term outcome of Lyme disease" (*Clinical Infectious Diseases,* vol. 31 [2000]: 1149–54), S. Varde's "Prevalence of tick-borne pathogens in Ixodes scapularis in a rural New Jersey county" (*Emerging Infectious Diseases,* vol. 4 [1998]: 97–99), E. K. Hofmeister's "Cosegregation of a novel Bartonella species with *Borrelia burgdorferi* and *Babesia microti* in *Peromyscus leukopus*" (*Journal of Infectious Diseases,* vol. 177 [1998]: 409–16), Johann Bakken's "Serological evidence of human granulocytic ehrlichiosis in Norway" (*European Journal of Clinical Microbiology and Infectious Diseases,* vol. 15 [1996]: 829–32), I. Christova's "Human granulocytic ehrlichiosis in Bulgaria" (*American Journal of Tropical Medicine and Hygiene,* vol. 60 [1999]: 58–61), Steve Dumler's "A population-based seroepidemiologic study of human granulocytic ehrlichiosis and Lyme borreliosis on the west coast of Sweden" (*Journal of Infectious Diseases,* vol. 175 [1997]: 720–22), N. Pusterla's "Serological evidence of human granulocytic ehrlichiosis in Switzerland" (*European Journal of Clinical Microbiology and Infectious Diseases,* vol. 17 [1998]: 207–9), and Gary Wormser's "Positive Lyme disease serology in patients with clinical and laboratory evidence of human granulocytic ehrlichiosis" (*American Journal of Clinical Pathology,* vol. 107 [1997]: 142–47).

CHAPTER 21 • CRACKS IN THE THEORY

I interviewed Drs. Ed Masters (telephone, 1994, 2000, 2001), Brian Fallon (telephone, 2001), Ken Leigner (telephone, 1994), James Oliver (telephone, 2001), and Grant Campbell (of the CDC, 2001) and used material from a letter from Dr. Masters to me (2000). I also used some material from Polly Murray's book (Chapter 1) and the interview with Joe Dowhan (Chapter 10). Several articles written by Ed Masters and/or H. Denny Donnell were helpful: Masters, "Erythema migrans in the South" (*Archives of Internal Medicine,* vol. 158 [1998]: 2162–65); Masters and Donnell, "Epidemiologic and diagnostic studies of patients with suspected early Lyme disease Missouri, 1990–1993" (letter to the editor, *Journal of Infectious Diseases,* vol. 173 [1996]: 1527–28); Masters and Donnell, "Lyme and/or Lyme-like disease in Missouri," (*Missouri Medicine,* vol. 92 [1995]: 346–53); and Donnell, "Erythema chronicum migrans, ticks and Lyme disease in Missouri" (*Missouri Medicine,* vol. 96 [1999]: 476). The above letter to the editor was in response to an article by Grant Campbell in 1995 titled "Epidemiologic and diagnostic studies of patients with suspected early Lyme disease, Missouri, 1990–1993" in the *Journal of Infectious Diseases* (vol. 172: 470–80). Alan Barbour described a possible tick pathogen for these southern cases in 1996 in the *Journal of Infectious Diseases*, "Identification of an uncultivatable Borrelia species in the hard tick *Amblyomma americanum:* possible agent of a Lyme-like illness" (vol. 173: 403–9). One of the best overviews of Lyme disease in the south was written by James Oliver in the *Journal of Parisitology* in 1996, "Lyme borreliosis in the southern United States: a review" (vol. 82: 926–35).

I also viewed the videotape and quoted from the official transcript of the U.S. Senate hearings on Lyme disease (*Lyme Disease: A Diagnostic and Treatment Dilemma*) held in August 1993 and sponsored by Senator Ted Kennedy and the Labor and Human Resources Committee. The transcript was printed by the U.S. Government Printing Office in Washington, D.C. I read several articles by Brian Fallon and colleagues: "The neuropsychiatric manifestations of Lyme Borreliosis" (*Psychiatric Quarterly*, vol. 63 [1992]: 95–117), "Psychiatric manifestations of Lyme Borreliosis" (*Journal of Clinical Psychiatry*, vol. 54 [1993]: 263–68), "Lyme disease: a neuropsychiatric illness" (*American Journal of Psychiatry*, vol. 151 [1994]: 1571–83), "Acute disseminated encephalomyelitis" (*Journal of Neuropsychiatry and Clinical Neurosciences*, vol. 10 [1998]: 366–67), and "The underdiagnosis of neuropsychiatric Lyme disease in children and adults" (*Psychiatric Clinics of North America*, vol. 21 [1998]: 693–703). Ken Leigner's article "Recurrent erythema migrans despite extended antibiotic treatment with minocycline in a patient with persisting *Borrelia burgdorferi* infection" (*Journal of the American Academy of Dermatology*, vol. 28 [1993]: 312–14) was also helpful.

CHAPTER 22 • ANOTHER PARADIGM

I quote from three books that I personally found fascinating reading and recommend to others: Dava Sobel's *Galileo's Daughter* (New York: Penguin Books, 2000); Thomas Kuhn's *The Structure of Scientific Revolutions* (2nd ed., Chicago: University of Chicago Press, 1970), a book I first enjoyed while in college before Lyme disease had been so named; and the book edited by K. Codell Carter on I. Semmelweis's *The Etiology, Concept, and Prophylaxis of Childbed Fever* (Madison: University of Wisconsin Press, 1983), which made excellent reading. While well into my book, David Grann published an article, "Stalking Doctor Steere," in the *New York Times Sunday Magazine* (June 17, 2001, pages 52–57). Grann spoke directly with Steere, and I found this article quite good. I also used information from the aforementioned U.S. Senate hearings transcript (Chapter 21). Two studies about overdiagnosis that I discuss are by Leonard Sigal, "Summary of the first 100 patients seen at a Lyme disease referral center" (*American Journal of Medicine*, vol. 88 [1990]: 577–81), and Steere, "The over-diagnosis of Lyme disease" (*JAMA*, vol. 269 [1993]: 1812–16). Three other useful articles are Ruth Montgomery's "The fate of Borrelia burgdorferi, the agent for Lyme disease, in mouse macrophages: destruction, survival, recovery" (*Journal of Immunology*, vol. 150 [1993]: 909–915), Hans-Walter Pfister's "Latent Lyme neuroborreliosis: presence of *Borrelia burgdorferi* in the cerebrospinal fluid without concurrent inflammatory signs" (*Neurology,* vol. 39 [1989]: 118–20), and Kostis Georgilis's "Fibroblasts protect the Lyme disease spirochete, Borrelia burgdorferi from ceftriaxone in vitro" (*Journal of Infectious Diseases,* vol. 166 [1992]: 440–44).

CHAPTER 23 • THERAPEUTIC ADVENTURES

A document available on the Web site of Dr. Joseph Burrascano (http://dwp. bigplanet.com/eojlyme) was useful: the eighth edition of his "Managing Lyme disease—diagnostic hints and treatment guidelines for Lyme Borreliosis" (copyright June 1993). I used three articles that address complications from prolonged antibiotic therapy for Lyme disease: M. Eckman's "Cost effectiveness of oral as compared with intravenous antibiotic therapy for patients with early Lyme disease or Lyme arthritis" (*New England Journal of Medicine,* vol. 337 [1997]: 357–63), P. J. Ettestad's "Biliary complications in the treatment of unsubstantiated Lyme disease" (*Journal of Infectious Diseases,* vol. 171 [1995]: 356–61), and R. Patel's "Death from inappropriate therapy for Lyme disease" (*Clinical Infectious Diseases,* vol. 31 [2000]: 1107–9).

I read a number of entries from Lora Mermin's compilation of articles and testimonials about Lyme disease called *Lyme Disease 1991: Patient/Physician Perspectives from the U.S. and Canada* (Madison, Wisc.: Lyme Disease Education Project, 1992). The experience of Craig Walker and his daughter with malariatherapy comes from this source. Henry Heimlich published a letter, "Should we try malariotherapy for Lyme disease?," in the *New England Journal of Medicine* in 1990 (vol. 322: 1234–35). Two articles that deal with the origins of malariatherapy are J. Wagner von Jauregg's landmark article "The treatment of general paresis by inoculation of malaria," published in the *Journal of Nervous and Mental Diseases* (vol. 55 [1922]: 369–75), and H. Delgado's "Treatment of paresis by inoculations with malaria" in the same journal (vol. 55 [1922]: 376–89). Historical accounts of the actual use of malariatherapy in more modern times include Eli Chernin's "The malariatherapy of neurosyphilis" (*Journal of Parasitology,* vol. 70 [1984]: 611–17) and Jeffrey Sartin's "From mercury to penicillin: the history of treatment of syphilis at the Mayo Clinic, 1916–1955" (*Journal of the American Academy of Dermatology,* vol. 32 [1995]: 255–61). Heimlich's more recent work on malariatherapy, mostly used for HIV infection, include "Malariotherapy for HIV patients" (*Mechanics of Ageing and Development,* vol. 93 [1997]: 79–85) and "Malaria therapy: the value of a randomized controlled trial" (*JAMA,* vol. 269 [1993]: 211–12). Two reports by the CDC on this therapy can be found in *Morbidity and Mortality Weekly Report* ("Epidemiologic notes and reports: imported malaria associated with malariatherapy of Lyme disease—New Jersey," vol. 39 [1990], and "Update: self-induced malaria associated with malariotherapy for Lyme disease—Texas," vol. 40 [1991]). An additional reference is Charles Pavia's "Preliminary in vitro and in vivo findings of hyperbaric oxygen treatment in experimental Bb infections," an oral presentation at the Thirteenth International Scientific Conference on Lyme Disease and Other Tick-Borne Disorders held in Hartford, Connecticut, in 2000 (this is a different series of conferences than the two mentioned in the book; this one is sponsored by the Lyme Disease Foundation).

CHAPTER 24 • GENOMES AND VACCINES

Much of the information about the work of James Watson and Francis Crick comes from the Nobel Prize Web site (mentioned above, Chapter 12), as well as the landmark article that they co-wrote and was published in the April 1953 issue of *Nature* ("A structure for deoxyribonucleic acid," vol. 171: 737–39). The data about the discovery of the entire genome of *B. burgdorferi* largely draw from a telephone interview with Dr. Claire Fraser in 2001 and two articles that she and co-workers wrote: "Genomic sequence of a Lyme disease spirochaete, *Borrelia burgdorferi*" (*Nature*, vol. 390 [1997]: 580–86) and "Complete genome sequence of *Treponema pallidum*, the syphilis spirochete" (*Science*, vol. 281 [1998]: 375–88). I also used an article by Dr. M. Pizza about the practical uses of genomic sequencing, "Identification of vaccine candidates against serogroup B meningococcus by whole-genome sequencing" (*Science*, vol. 287 [2000]: 1816–20).

The historical information about Jenner's work on vaccination and the role of Lady Montagu comes from the book by Meyer Friedman and Gerald Friedland (Chapter 8) on *Medicine's Ten Greatest Discoveries*. The quotation from Lady Montagu's writings is from the Internet Modern History Sourcebook at http://www.fordham.edu/halsall/mod/montagu-smallpox.html. Information about Louis Pasteur comes from the *Morbidity and Mortality Weekly Report* of July 5, 1985 ("Historical Perspectives, a centennial celebration: Pasteur and the modern era of immunization," vol. 34: 389–90) and a book by Hilaire Cuny, *Louis Pasteur: The Man and His Theories* (Greenwich: Fawcett Publications, 1963).

Early articles on the Lyme vaccine include D. Keller's "Safety and immunogenicity of a recombinant outer surface A Lyme vaccine" (*JAMA*, vol. 271 [1994]: 1764–68) and Robert Schoen's "Safety and immunogenicity of an outer surface protein A vaccine in subjects with previous Lyme disease" (*Journal of Infectious Diseases*, vol. 172 [1995]: 1324–29). The two major publications regarding clinical testing of the Osp A vaccine were published in the same issue of the *New England Journal of Medicine* (vol. 339: 209–22) in 1998. The first was by Allen Steere et al. ("Vaccination against Lyme disease with recombinant Borrelia burgdorferi outer-surface lipoprotein A with adjuvant") and the second by Leonard Sigal et al. ("A vaccine consisting of recombinant Borrelia burgdorferi outer-surface protein A to prevent Lyme disease"). Dr. Ferrieri's comments were taken from the transcript of the May 1998 FDA advisory committee meeting (Center for Biologics Evaluation and Research Advisory Committee, chaired by Dr. Ferrieri), which can be found in its entirety on the FDA Web site at http://fda.gov.

CHAPTER 25 • LEGAL AND POLITICAL BATTLES

I reviewed transcripts of other FDA advisory committee meetings, in January and November of 2001 (also available in their entirety on the FDA Web site, see above, Chapter 24), for quotations from Karen Forschner and Dr. Sidney Wolfe (of the Public Citizen's Health Research Group). These two meetings and the one mentioned in Chapter 24 took place in Bethesda, Maryland. I also reviewed an article by S. Lathrop published in *Vaccine* in 2002 (vol. 20: 1603–8) called "Adverse event reports following vaccination for Lyme disease: December 1998–July 2000." In 2002, I interviewed Dr. Ned Hayes of the CDC by telephone, who supplied perspective on this process. Although I did not include specific information from these interviews, I also spoke with two of the doctors who participated in the phase four studies of the Lyme disease vaccine—Drs. Arnold Chan and Richard Platt, both of Boston—in order to better understand those studies.

Concerning the legal issues surrounding Lyme disease, I spoke with Ira Maurer in 1999 and 2001 and with Stephen Sheller in 2002 about their involvement with lawsuits arising from Lyme disease and its treatment. Some of the information about the serologic findings and side effects of the Osp A vaccine comes from articles by Paul Fawcett and his group: "Arthritis following recombinant Osp A vaccination for Lyme disease" (*Journal of Rheumatology,* vol. 28 [2001]: 2555–57), "Effects of immunization with recombinant Osp A on serologic tests for Lyme borreliosis" (*Clinics in Diagnostic and Laboratory Immunology,* vol. 8 [2001]: 79–84), and "Comparison of immunodot and western blot assays for diagnosing Lyme borreliosis (*Clinics in Diagnostic and Laboratory Immunology,* vol. 5 [1998]: 503–6). The data surrounding the FDA and the drug Lotronex come from Robert Horton's piece in the May 19, 2001, issue of *Lancet* called "Lotronex and the FDA: a fatal erosion in integrity" (vol. 357: 1544–45; as well as some follow-up commentary that appeared in the August 4, 2001, issue). I spoke with Dr. Sam Donta, of Boston, in 1994 and 2001 for his views on the treatment of late-stage Lyme disease and the vaccine-induced side effects.

I also read and quote statistics from the 2002 *JAMA* article by N. Choudhry called "Relationships between authors of clinical practice guidelines and the pharmaceutical industry" (vol. 287: 612–17). The practice guideline for Lyme disease was written by a group of individuals (G. Wormser et al.) and was published as "Practice guidelines for the treatment of Lyme disease. The Infectious Diseases Society of America" (*Clinical Infectious Diseases,* vol. 31 [suppl, 2000]: 1–14). The information about the controversy surrounding Drs. Steere and Burrascano come from several sources. The best, and one that is worth reading for anyone interested in this aspect of the story, is the aforementioned article from the *New York Times Sunday Magazine* by David Grann (Chapter 22). I also accessed the Massachusetts Lyme Disease Coalition's Web site in 2001 (http://www.lymealliance.org/latest/steere.php) and obtained information from the Massachusetts Board of Registration in Medicine.

CHAPTER 26 · AN INDEPENDENT REALITY

Randy Shilts's book *And the Band Played On* covers the AIDS epidemic superbly (New York: St. Martins Press, 1987). I discuss information from a large study by Mark Klempner, published in 2001 in the *New England Journal of Medicine* (vol. 245: 85–92) and a response from Sam Donta in the same journal (vol. 345: 1424–25). Donta refers to his article in *Clinical Infectious Diseases* called "Tetracycline therapy for chronic Lyme disease" (vol. 25 [suppl, 1997]: S52–S56).

Regarding issues around the definition of Lyme disease and the relationship of Lyme disease to erythema migrans, I read J. Melski's "Language, logic and Lyme disease," a 1999 editorial in the *Archives of Dermatology* (vol. 135: 1398–1400). The same theme played out at the Ninth International Conference on Lyme Borreliosis and Other Tick-Borne Diseases held in New York City in August 2002, especially during presentations by Drs. Sam Telford and Alan Barbour. I read Steve Malawista's "Resolution of Lyme arthritis, acute or prolonged: a new look" (*Inflammation*, vol. 24 [2000]: 493–504) and listened to his presentation at the 2002 meetings in New York.

HIGHLIGHTED REFERENCES

Some readers may have become sufficiently interested in Lyme disease, its history, or some of the other subjects related to scientific inquiry that this book encompasses to want to know more. I therefore highlight here some of the sources, with brief comments, that such a reader might find particularly interesting and rewarding.

Polly Murray, *The Widening Circle* (New York: St. Martins Press, 1996). Mrs. Murray covers the history of the disease, largely from the perspective of one individual.

John Snow, *Snow on Cholera—Being a Reprint of Two Papers*, edited by William Frost (New York: The Commonwealth Fund, 1936). This readable classic in epidemiology is highly recommended and a "must-read" for those interested in that field.

For readers who like to turn to original scientific papers, the original report by Allen Steere and Steve Malawista, "Lyme arthritis: an epidemic of oligoarticular arthritis in children and adults in three Connecticut communities" (*Arthritis and Rheumatism*, vol. 20 [1977]: 7–17), makes good reading. The same can be said of the original report of Willy Burgdorfer et al. in *Science* of the discovery of the causal spirochete ("Lyme disease—a tick-borne spirochetosis?," vol. 216 [1982]: 1317–19).

The history of Lyme disease in Europe includes far more details than I chose to highlight in this book. Readers who want a more detailed account will enjoy the chapter "History of Lyme borreliosis in Europe," written by Drs. Klaus Weber and Hans-Walter Pfister, in the book *Aspects of Lyme Borreliosis*, edited by Weber and Willy Burgdorfer (Berlin: Springer-Verlag, 1992). The other chapter that makes compelling reading is written by Burgdorfer and is called "The historical road to the discovery of *B. burgdorferi*."

The April 2002 issue of *Medical Clinics of North America* is devoted to tick-borne diseases, including Lyme disease. The edition (vol. 86) was edited by Jonathan Edlow and published by Saunders (Philadelphia).

Alan Barbour, *Lyme Disease: The Cause, the Cure, the Controversy* (Baltimore: Johns Hopkins University Press, 1996). This highly recommended book is designed for the general reader. The chapter on serologic testing is especially lucid.

James Oliver has a large perspective on Lyme disease or the Lyme-like disease that is occurring in the southern United States. His piece "Lyme borreliosis in the southern United States: a review" in the *Journal of Parisitology* in 1996 (vol. 82: 926–

35) gives a clear, if technical, account of that situation. Another article, this one by Ed Masters, that makes a good companion piece is "Erythema migrans in the south," published in the *Archives of Internal Medicine* in 1998 (vol. 158: 2162–65).

Of the controversy surrounding Lyme disease, one source that is worth seeing is the transcript *Lyme Disease: A Diagnostic and Treatment Dilemma* from the U.S. Senate hearings held on August 5, 1993 and sponsored by Senator Ted Kennedy and the Labor and Human Resources Committee. The U.S. Government Printing Office in Washington, D.C., printed the entire transcript.

Dava Sobel, *Galileo's Daughter* (New York: Penguin Books, 2000). This was one of my favorite books that I read in preparation for writing *Bull's-Eye* and is a classic in terms of seeing science in its cultural context. Sobel tells the story of Galileo largely through the voice of his daughter.

Thomas S. Kuhn, *The Structure of Scientific Revolutions* (Chicago: University of Chicago Press, 1970). This book is similar in scope to Sobel's but is far more technical. It has become a classic text in the field of scientific inquiry.

To remind us of our past, and how ideas change through time, I recommend J. Sartin's "From mercury to penicillin: the history of treatment of syphilis at the Mayo Clinic—1916–1955," which was published in 1995 in the *Journal of the American Academy of Dermatology* (vol. 32: 255–61). Ideas change, and what is held dear to one generation may become the next generation's folly.

Although covering a different disease, the AIDS epidemic, Randy Shilts's book *And the Band Played On* (New York: St. Martins Press, 1987) is superb. This book also reminds us that we are not too "modern" to be affected by culture and context as regards our science.

Karen Vanderhoof-Forschner, *Everything You Need to Know About Lyme Disease* (New York: John Wiley and Sons, 1997). Recommended for readers who wish to read a book that is written by someone who sees the controversies of Lyme disease from the perspective of the alternative camp.

Arno Karlen, *Biography of a Germ* (New York: Pantheon Books, 2000). This book is a fanciful but information-packed story about the spirochete *B. burgdorferi.*

ACA: See *acrodermatitis chronicum atrophicans.*

acrodermatitis chronicum atrophicans: The chronic skin lesion of Lyme disease, found in European patients and first described in 1883.

Amblyomma: A genus of hard tick, associated with some forms of ehrlichiosis and Masters' disease (or southern tick-associated rash illness [STARI]).

antibody: A protein manufactured by lymphocytes that help to fight infections by invading microorganisms (such as bacteria or viruses).

antigen: The portion of an invading microorganism (bacteria or virus) to which an antibody binds.

arthritis: A general term for inflammation of a joint, sometimes also called *synovitis.* The condition could be caused by crystals (gouty arthritis), bacteria (septic arthritis), or other things (for example, rheumatoid arthritis).

arthrocentesis: A diagnostic medical procedure to aspirate fluid from an inflamed or injured joint.

babesiosis: A tick-borne disease (of both animals and humans) characterized by fevers and chills.

Bannwarth's syndrome: An inflammatory disease of the central nervous system found predominantly in Europe and which is one manifestation of Lyme disease.

Bell's palsy: Paralysis of half of the face due to inflammation of the facial nerve. This condition has many causes, among which is Lyme disease.

Borrelia: A genus of bacteria that belongs to the spirochetes. The agents that cause relapsing fever and Lyme disease are borreliae.

Borrelia afzelii: The species of *Borrelia* that causes some cases of Lyme disease in Europe, especially cases of acrodermatitis chronicum atrophicans.

Borrelia burgdorferi: The causative agent of Lyme disease. *Borrelia burgdorferi* sensu lato refers to the group of bacteria including *Borrelia burgdorferi* sensu stricto (the cause of U.S. and some European cases of Lyme disease), *Borrelia afzelii,* and *Borrelia garinii* (the causes of the remainder of European cases).

Borrelia garinii: The species of *Borrelia* that causes some cases of Lyme disease in Europe, especially cases with neurological involvement.

ceftriaxone: A powerful intravenous antibiotic used to treat Lyme disease.

cellulitis: An infection, usually caused by staphylococcus or streptococcus bacteria, of the skin. This can be confused with EM.

Colorado tick fever: An illness found in the western United States caused by a tick-borne virus.

Coxiella burnetii: The microorganism responsible for Q fever, a rickettsial disease. This was the disease that Willy Burgdorfer started investigating at the beginning of his career in Switzerland.

Dermacentor: A genus of ticks that includes the tick that is the vector of Rocky Mountain spotted fever.

Dermacentor andersoni: The tick vector of Rocky Mountain spotted fever and Colorado tick fever in the western United States.

Dermacentor variabilis: The tick vector of Rocky Mountain spotted fever in the eastern United States.

doxycycline: A tetracycline-group antibiotic that is useful for treating Lyme disease and ehrlichiosis.

ECM: See *erythema chronicum migrans.*

ehrlichiosis: A group of tick-borne diseases characterized by fevers, chills, and sometimes rash.

ELISA: Acronym for enzyme-linked immunosorbent assay, a test for antibodies against *B. burgdorferi* in a patient's serum. Because the test is automated, scientists hoped it would replace the IFA; however, the ELISA has a high level of false-positive results.

erythema chronicum migrans (ECM): The rash of early Lyme disease. This term, first coined by Lipschutz in his 1913 report, was used during the early years of Lyme disease but has gradually been replaced by the term erythema migrans (EM), which has priority and is the preferred term.

EM: See *erythema migrans.*

erythema migrans (EM): The rash of early Lyme disease. This term was first coined by Arvid Afzelius in 1910 and is preferred to the term erythema chronicum migrans (ECM).

Garin-Bujadoux-Bannwarth's syndrome: The syndrome of neurological involvement of the nerve roots and sometimes the meninges. Originally described in Europe, first by Garin and Bujadoux and later by Bannwarth.

gout: A disease of uric acid metabolism that can lead to acute arthritis.

IFA: Acronym for immunofluorescent assay, a test for antibodies again *B. burgdorferi* in a patient's serum. Each test must be interpreted by a laboratory technician, which makes it labor- and time-intensive. This was the first diagnostic test used for Lyme disease in the 1980s.

Ixodes: A genus of hard ticks that includes the species responsible for Lyme disease.

Ixodes dammini: Thought to be the species of tick that is the vector for *Borrelia burgdorferi* in the northeastern United States. Subsequent research showed this not to be a separate tick species, but actually the same as *Ixodes scapularis.*

Ixodes pacificus: The tick vector for *Borrelia burgdorferi* in the northwestern United States.

Ixodes ricinus: The tick vector for *Borrelia burgdorferi* (and related *Borrelia*) in much of Europe.

Ixodes scapularis: The tick vector for *Borrelia burgdorferi* in the eastern United States.

JRA: See *juvenile rheumatoid arthritis.*

juvenile rheumatoid arthritis: An uncommon form of arthritis found mostly in children that was the leading diagnosis in many of the children in Lyme, Connecticut, before the discovery of Lyme disease.

lumbar puncture: A diagnostic medical procedure to remove cerebrospinal fluid (the fluid that bathes the brain and spinal cord) out of the spinal canal. Sometimes also called a spinal tap.

lymphocyte: A kind of white blood cell. One type of lymphocyte, called a B cell, makes antibodies.

Masters' disease: A Lyme-like disease found in the southeastern and midcentral United States, also called southern tick-associated rash illness (STARI) by the Centers for Disease Control and Prevention.

meningitis: Inflammation of the meninges, the covering layer of the brain and spinal cord. Meningitis can be caused by viruses and bacteria, including the Lyme disease spirochete.

Ornithodoros: The genus of ticks that is the vector of relapsing fever.

polyradiculitis: Inflammation of multiple nerve roots and one neurological manifestation of Lyme disease.

Q fever: A (sometimes) tick-borne disease characterized by fevers. It is caused by *Coxiella burnetii.*

radiculitis: Inflammation of nerve roots (radicles) that exit the spinal cord.

relapsing fever: A tick-borne (and also louse-borne) disease caused by various *Borrelia* species, characterized by recurrent bouts of fevers.

RMSF: See *Rocky Mountain spotted fever.*

Rocky Mountain spotted fever (RMSF): A tick-borne disease caused by the organism *Rickettsia rickettsia,* characterized by fevers and rash.

serologic testing for Lyme disease: Blood tests that measure antibodies to *Borrelia burgdorferi.* These tests do not prove or disprove the diagnosis; as indirect tests, they must be interpreted in a clinical context.

spirochete: A kind of bacteria shaped like a corkscrew. *Borrelia* are a type of spirochete.

STARI: See Masters' disease.

synovial biopsy: A diagnostic medical procedure by which a physician obtains a small piece of synovium so that it can be examined in the laboratory.

synovium: The tissue that lines the joints of the body.

Treponema pallidum: The agent that causes syphilis. This spirochete can still not be cultured on artificial medium in the laboratory.

Treponeme: A class of spirochete.

Western blot: A blood test for Lyme disease that measures specific antibodies against *Borrelia burgdorferi.* This test is usually used as a back-up test for patients whose ELISA tests are positive or equivocal.

yellow fever: The viral, mosquito-transmitted disease for which Walter Reed and his colleagues performed self-experimentation while working in Cuba.

Note: The abbreviation LD is used to indicate Lyme disease throughout index.

INDEX

Ackerman, Rudolph, 126–28, 127(photo), 138, 248
acrodermatitis chronica atrophicans (ACA), 68–71, 94, 124, 144, 183
Afzelius, Arvid, 55–57, 146
alternative view of LD, 196–97, 204–11, 212–14, 220. *See also* antibiotics; controversy over LD
Amblyomma americanum (Lone Star tick), 159, 184, 185(photo), 191–92, 256(table)
Anderson, John, 90, 91(photo), 92–94, 97, 99, 128, 139, 248
Andiman, Warren, 44
And the Band Played On (Shilts), 244
anthrax, 107, 228, 250
antibiotics: bacterial resistance, 112–13; and coinfection, 185–86; duration, 194, 195–97, 205, 207–8, 210–11, 212–14, 244–45; effectiveness, 119–20, 144, 193; EM treated, 50, 52, 66, 68, 73–74, 79, 116; intravenous antibiotics, 144, 212–14, 239; trials, 110–12, 115–16; Yale team's initial skepticism, 73–74, 77, 79–80, 110
antibodies, 170–72. *See also* ELISA; IFA tests
arboviruses, 42–44
Aristotle, 84, 199
arthritis: after vaccination, 237; clustering, 27, 40 (*see also* geographical range of LD); in LD, 37–42, 115, 144, 255(table); types/causes, 12–14, 32–33, 43–45. *See also* joint pain and swelling; juvenile rheumatoid arthritis
Arthur, Don, 83–84

babesiosis, 63, 90–91, 93, 99–101, 117, 180–85, 256(table)
bacteria, 63–64, 66, 107–9, 112–13. *See also* antibiotics; borreliae; rickettsiae; spirochetes; ulcers
Bafverstedt, Bo, 69
Banks, Nathan, 146

Bannwarth, Alfred, 69–70. *See also* Bannwarth's syndrome
Bannwarth's syndrome, 69–70, 126–28
Barbour, Alan, 134(photo), 134–37, 142–43, 191–92
B. burgdorferi. See *Borrelia burgdorferi*
Bell's palsy, 5, 70, 77
Benach, Jorge, 90, 92(photo), 98–99, 128–30, 133–34, 137–38, 142–43, 248
Binder, Erich, 67, 68
birds, 155–56
blood banks, 243–44
blood tests. *See* laboratory testing
Borrelia burgdorferi, 137(photo); discovery, 134–40; earliest evidence, 147–48; genetic diversity, 183–84, 188–89; genome defined, 222–24; incubation period, 190; inhibited by high temperature, 220; nomenclature, 138, 142–43, 183–84; other syndromes triggered, 207, 208–10; outside the Northeast, 156, 159, 190; persistence, 197–98, 210–11 (*see also* controversy over LD); test development, 174, 224–25 (*see also* laboratory testing); vaccines, 229–30. *See also* borreliae; spirochetes
borreliae, 105; *B. duttonii,* 103, 106; considered as EM cause, 125–26; cross-reactivity, 122, 123; culturing methods, 109; diversity, 246. See also *Borrelia burgdorferi*; spirochetes
Buchwald, Alfred, 68–69
Bujadoux, Dr., 57–60, 126–27
bull's-eye rash. *See* erythema migrans
Burckhardt, Jean Louis, 69
Burgdorfer, Willy, 91(photo), 93(photo), 102, 104, 248; *B. burgdorferi* named for, 93, 142–43; doctoral thesis, 102–4; LD spirochete identified, 130–40; postgraduate career, 104–5; RMSF investigated, 90, 97–99

Burrascano, Joseph Jr., 204–5, 206–7, 212, 240, 249
Burrows, William, 47(photo), 48–54, 73, 75–76, 79–80, 247–48

CDC. *See* Centers for Disease Control and Prevention
cell membranes, 66, 120–21
cellulitis, 48–49
Centers for Disease Control and Prevention (CDC): and cases in nonendemic areas, 156–59, 189–91, 245–46; causal organism sought, 119; Dearborn criteria, 177–78; disease definition, 156–57, 159, 175, 245–46; EIS program, 18–19; J. Mensch's call to, 15–16; reporting of LD, 152–54, 156–57, 159; and transfusion-related AIDS, 244. *See also* investigation of LD
Chain, Ernst, 67
Chikungunya fever, 43
cholera, 20–23, 26, 67, 108, 250
chronic fatigue syndrome, 206, 208, 209, 210
classification, biological, 64–65, 84–85. *See also* nomenclature
coinfection, 180–87. *See also* babesiosis
Colorado tick fever, 105, 130, 256(table)
complexity of LD, 192–98
Connaught (pharmaceutical company), 229–30
Connecticut: clustering of cases, 1–11, 19–20, 24–25(maps), 27, 29–32, 36–42, 46–50, 52–54, 78, 81–83, 87–88; deer population, 151–53; public concern, 78–79; RMSF in, 97; ticks in, 81–83, 87–88, 128. *See also* geographical range of LD; Yale team's investigation; *specific individuals*
controversy over LD: cases in nonendemic areas, 156–59, 189–91, 245–46; conventional vs. alternative camps, 79–80, 189–98, 204–11,
212–14, 220, 240–42, 244–46; legal/political issues, 236–37, 239–42; vaccines, 229–30, 232, 234–37
conventional view of LD, 79–80, 192–98, 204–11, 239–41. *See also* controversy over LD
Copernicus, Nicolaus, 200, 202
Crick, Francis, 221–22

Dammin, Gustav, 56–57, 117
deer, 86(fig.), 89, 150–52, 156
deer tick. *See Ixodes scapularis*
depression, 10–11, 195, 209
Dermacentor genus, 83(photo), 85, 95, 96, 132, 146, 256(table). *See also* Rocky Mountain spotted fever; ticks
diagnosis: of arthritis, 13; coinfection, 180–87 (*see also* babesiosis); conventional vs. alternative camps, 205–8 (*see also* Masters' disease); generally, 3–4, 179–80; vector presence and, 117, 159. *See also* laboratory testing
dog tick (*D. variabilis*), 83(photo), 96, 132. *See also* Rocky Mountain spotted fever
Donnell, H. Denny, 189–90
Donta, Sam, 245
Dowhan, Joe, 82–83, 197–98, 250
Dumler, J. Stephen, 96
Dutton, Joseph, 106

ECM. *See* erythema migrans
Ehrlich, Paul, 216
ehrlichiosis, 180–81, 183, 184–86, 256(table), 257(table)
ELISA, 170–75, 237
EM. *See* erythema migrans
enzyme-linked immunosorbent assay (ELISA), 170–75, 237
erythema migrans (EM, ECM): antibiotics and, 50, 52, 66, 68, 73–74, 79, 116 (*see also* antibiotics); appearance, 7, 40, 53(photo), 55, 143; in

Europe, 51, 54, 55–61, 68–71, 123–28, 138 (*see also* Europe); nomenclature, 56, 60, 146–47; in the Northeast, 5, 7, 40–41, 46–54, 73, 75–77; outside the Northeast, 51–52, 92–93, 158–59, 246; spirochete suggested as cause, 61, 66–67, 104, 125–26; statistics, 205. *See also* symptoms of LD

Europe: contemporary research, 123–28, 183–84, 188–89; deer population, 152; history of EM/LD, 51, 54, 55–61, 66, 68–71, 126–28, 146–47; range of LD, 138, 149; U.S. vs. European manifestations, 144. See also *Ixodes* genus: *I. ricinus*

facial paralysis, 5, 70, 77
Fallon, Brian, 194–95, 245, 249
Fawcett, Paul, 177–78, 237
Ferrieri, Patricia, 230, 236
fibromyalgia, 206, 207–8, 209, 210
First International Symposium on LD, 141–44
Florey, Howard, 67
Food and Drug Administration (FDA), 232–35, 238–39
Forshner, Karen and son, 193–94, 234, 236, 249
Fraser, Claire, 222, 223–24

Galileo Galilei, 200–201
Galileo's Daughter (Sobel), 200
Garin, Charles, 57–60, 126–27
Geigy, Rudolph, 102–3
geographical range of LD: clustering in the Northeast, 1–7, 11–12, 24–25(maps), 26–27, 30–31, 40, 42, 78–80, 81–82, 87–88, 128–29 (*see also* Connecticut; New York); and coinfection, 182–84; expansion, 145, 155–59; historical range, 96–97, 147–49; outside the Northeast, 117, 154–59, 189–92, 245–46; U.S. vs. European manifestations, 144.

See also Connecticut; Europe; New York
Georgia, 156–57, 159
germ theory, 202–3
Gifford, Robert (Bob), 8, 29, 31
GlaxoSmithKline (SmithKline Beecham), 229–30, 231–32, 238, 249
Gotz, Hans, 70
Grunwaldt, Edgar, 54, 90–91, 101, 130, 137

Haas, Victor, 104
Hanrahan, John, 128–29
Hansen, Thomas, 51
Harden, Victoria, 95–96
Hartmann, Kuno, 69
Haverhill fever, 44–45
Hayes, Ned, 233
heart complications, 77, 144
Heimlich, Henry, 214, 220
Hellerstrom, Sven, 51, 60–61, 66, 104
hemolymph test, 103
Herxheimer, Karl, 69
HGE and HME. *See* ehrlichiosis
Horstrup, Peter, 126–28
Horton, Richard, 238–39
human immunodeficiency virus (HIV), 63, 243–44

I. dammini. See Ixodes scapularis
IFA tests, 120–23, 133–35, 136(fig.), 169
immune system: antibodies, 120–23, 170–72 (*see also* laboratory testing); autoimmune disorders, 209; and inflammatory illness, 34–35. *See also* vaccines
immunofluorescent antibody tests. *See* IFA tests
incubation period of LD, 190
insects and other arthropods, as disease vectors, 42–43, 85–87. *See also* mosquitoes; *headings beginning with* tick

investigation of LD: biases, 73–75; blind men and elephant metaphor, 72–74; causal organism sought, 44, 75–76, 99–100, 118–29, 130–40 (see also *Borrelia burgdorferi*); and coinfection, 181–84; cracks in the theory, 188–98; international symposium, 141–44; methods, 23, 24–25(maps), 26–27, 37–39, 75–76 (*see also* laboratory testing); psychiatric symptoms explored, 194–95; Senate hearings, 193–94, 206–7; virus believed cause, 44, 75–76, 126–28. *See also* Yale team's investigation

I. ricinus. See Ixodes genus
I. scapularis. See Ixodes scapularis
Ixodes genus, 85, 117, 139, 256(table); *I. ricinus* (sheep tick), 55, 57, 94, 104, 126, 131–32, 139. See also *Ixodes scapularis*; ticks
Ixodes scapularis (*I. dammini*; deer tick), 83(photo), 85–87; LD connection suspected, 81–83, 87–89, 99–100; life cycle, 86(fig.), 151, 156; nomenclature, 117, 145–46; other diseases transmitted, 117, 181–83, 256(table) (*see also* babesiosis); population, 151, 155; range, 146, 155–57. See also *Borrelia burgdorferi*; ticks

Jarisch-Herxheimer reaction, 119–20
Jenner, Edward, 225–27
Johnson, Russ, 142–43
joint pain and swelling: after treatment, 209; case histories, 1–2, 5, 9–12, 15, 57–59, 69, 193; patterns, 39, 40–42, 76–77; treatment guidelines, 80. *See also* arthritis; fibromyalgia; juvenile rheumatoid arthritis
JRA. *See* juvenile rheumatoid arthritis
juvenile rheumatoid arthritis (JRA), 6–7, 10–12, 14–15, 26–27, 30–31, 41–42. *See also* arthritis

Kalm, Pehr, 84
Kelly, Richard, 109, 224
Koch, Robert, 21, 106–9; Koch's postulates, 108, 133, 138
Kuhn, Thomas S., 201–2, 243

laboratory testing: accuracy, 160–69, 170, 173–78, 237; cross-reactivity, 122, 123, 172–74, 184; ELISA, 170–75, 237; IFA tests, 120–23, 133–35, 136(fig.), 169; interpretation, 190; PCR test, 147–49; timing, 168, 174–75; Western blot test, 170, 175–78, 237
Lea, John, 21
legal issues of LD, 236–37, 239–40
Leigner, Kenneth, 196–97, 211
Lennhoff, Carl, 62, 64, 65–66, 104
leptospires and leptospirosis, 120
Linnaeus, Carolus, 64–65
Lipschutz, Benjamin, 56, 57, 60, 146
Lone Star tick (*A. americanum*), 159, 184, 185(photo), 191–92, 256 (table)
Lotronex, 238–39
Lyme, Connecticut, area. *See* Connecticut
Lyme Disease 1991 (Mermin), 214
LYMErix (vaccine), 229–30, 231–37, 249
lymphocytoma, 69–71, 94, 144

Magnarelli, Louis, 90, 91(photo), 97, 99, 128, 139
malaria, 43, 63, 219
malariatherapy, 214–15, 217–20
Malawista, Stephen, 30(photo), 116, 248, 250; and the international symposium, 144; Yale investigation, 30, 32, 37, 73–75, 77–78, 117 (*see also* Yale team's investigation)
Marshall, Barry, 35, 113–14, 203–4
Mast, William, 46–48, 47(photo), 52–54, 73, 79–80, 247–48

Masters' disease, 158–59, 185(photo), 245–46, 256(table). *See also* Masters, Ed

Masters, Ed, 157(photo), 157–59, 189–91, 246, 248–49

Maurer, Ira, 239

meningitis, 58–60, 69–70, 77, 125, 144, 225, 255(table). *See also* neurological symptoms

Mensch, Judith and family, 9–12, 15–16, 19, 29, 81, 151, 247

Mermin, Lora, 214

mice, 86(fig.), 89, 93, 152, 156

Missouri, 157–59, 189–91. *See also* Masters' disease

Montague, Lady Mary Wortley, 225–26

mosquitoes, 43, 67–68. *See also* malaria

Mullis, Kary, 148

Murray, Polly and family, 1–8, 2(photo), 19, 31–32, 81, 141–42, 192–94, 247

neurological symptoms, 5, 39–40, 70, 74, 77, 143–44, 208–10, 255(table). See also *specific conditions and symptoms*

New York: LD in, 54, 128–29, 132–33, 147, 155–56, 196–97; other diseases in, 90–91, 98–99, 101, 132–33

Nields, Jennifer, 194–95

nomenclature: *B. burgdorferi*, 138, 142–43, 183–84; and classification, 64–65; deer ticks, 117, 145–46; EM vs. ECM, 56, 60, 146–47; LD, 73–74, 77

Obermeier, Otto, 105

Oliver, James, 145, 157, 192

Ornithodorus genus, 85, 103

Osler, Sir William, 13, 96, 112, 215–16

paradigm shifts, 199–204, 243–44, 246–47

parasites, 63

Paschoud, Jean-Marie, 70

Pasteur, Louis, 227–29

Paterson family, 11–12

PCR test, 147–49

penicillin, 66–68, 116, 144, 185–86. *See also* antibiotics

Persing, David, 148

Pettenkofer, Max Josef Von, 21, 67, 108

pharmaceutical companies, 241. *See also* GlaxoSmithKline

polymerase chain reaction (PCR) test, 147–49

pregnancy and LD, 193–94

prions, 63, 204

psychiatric symptoms, 10–11, 194–95, 209, 255(table)

Ptolemy, Claudius, 199

rash. *See* acrodermatitis chronica atrophicans; erythema migrans; lymphocytoma

rat-bite fever, 44–45

Reed, Walter, 67–68

relapsing fever, 103–6, 109, 126, 246, 256(table)

Rensberger, Boyce, 78

reporting of LD, 152–54, 156–57, 159

rheumatic fever, 33–34, 209

Ricketts, Howard Taylor, 94–95, 96, 146

rickettsiae, 63–64, 97, 125, 131–32. *See also* Rocky Mountain spotted fever

Rocky Mountain spotted fever (RMSF), 64, 83(photo), 94–99, 130–33, 146, 256(table)

Ross River disease, 43–44

rotavirus vaccine, 235

Schmid, George, 119–20, 123, 154–55

Schur, Peter, 6

Scott, H. Harold, 21

Scrimenti, Rudolph, 51–52, 52(photo), 92–93
self-experimentation, 67–68, 70, 105, 114
Semmelweis, Ignaz, 202–3
sheep tick. See Ixodes genus
Sheller, Stephen, 236–37
Shilts, Randy, 244
Shope, Robert E., 44, 100
Sigal, Leonard, 205–6, 229–30
smallpox vaccine, 225–27, 228
Smith, Robert, 156
Smith, Theobald, 86–87
SmithKline Beecham. See GlaxoSmithKline
Snow, John, 20–23, 26, 108–9
Snydman, David, 17, 18(photo), 248; bias, 73–75; early investigations, 19–20, 23, 24–25(maps), 26–27, 32–33, 37; Steere contacted, 29–31. See also Yale team's investigation
Sobel, Dava, 200
Spielman, Andrew, 91, 101, 117, 145, 248
spinal tap, 58–59, 196
spirochetes, 62; difficulty culturing, 64, 105–6, 109, 118–19; diversity in Georgia, 157; hemolymph test developed, 103; Jarisch-Herxheimer reaction, 119–20; Lennhoff's work, 65–66; probable link to LD, 118–20; symptoms attributed to, 54, 61, 62, 93, 104; syphilis caused by, 64, 216 (see also syphilis). See also Borrelia burgdorferi; borreliae
stages of LD, 76–77, 117, 143–44; fetal infection, 193–94; non-standard symptoms/progression, 192–98; stage one, 143, 255(table); stage two, 143–44, 255(table); stage three, 144, 255(table); timing of tests, 168, 174–75. See also specific symptoms
Steere, Allen, 16, 19, 29, 248; antibiotic trials, 110–12, 115–16; bias, 73–75; Burgdorfer consulted, 131;

causal organism sought, 117, 118–20, 123; complaints against, 239–40; conventional camp upheld, 204, 206–7; and J. Dowhan, 82–83, 197–98; early investigations, 29–32, 37–39, 81, 151; and the international symposium, 141–43; and P. Murray, 31–32, 192–93; summer of 1976, 75–80, 82–83; vaccine tested, 229–30; virus believed cause, 75–76, 128. See also Yale team's investigation
Stiles, Charles, 146
Stoenner, Herbert, 109, 135
streptococcal infection (strep), 33, 167–68, 209. See also rheumatic fever
The Structure of Scientific Revolutions (Kuhn), 201–2, 243
support groups, 193, 194, 205
surveillance, active vs. passive, 154–56
symptoms of LD, 39–40; after vaccination, 232, 237; coinfection and, 182, 184; nonstandard symptoms/progression, 179, 192–98; patterns, 39, 40–42, 76–77; persistence, 197–98, 205–11; and stages, 143–44, 255(table). See also arthritis; erythema migrans; joint pain and swelling; juvenile rheumatoid arthritis; neurological symptoms; psychiatric symptoms; specific individuals
syphilis, 59, 64, 103, 168, 215–18

temporal range of LD, 27, 40–41, 82, 96–97, 147–54
Texas cattle fever, 85–87, 95, 257(table)
Thompson, Robert, 105
Thyresson, Nils, 66, 70
tick bites: EM caused, 51–52, 55, 57–60, 94 (see also erythema migrans); LD connection made, 81–83, 87–

88; noticed by patients, 55, 57, 61, 81–83, 88, 159. *See also* tick-borne diseases; ticks

tick-borne diseases, 256–57(table); coinfection, 180–87; Colorado tick fever, 105, 130, 256(table); in Europe (*see* Europe); 1970 milestones, 92–94; relapsing fever, 103–6, 109, 126, 246, 256(table); Texas cattle fever, 86–87, 95, 257(table); transmission mechanism, 186. *See also* babesiosis; ehrlichiosis; erythema migrans; Rocky Mountain spotted fever; tick bites; ticks; *specific LD topics*

ticks, 83–85, 103; *A. americanum* (Lone Star tick), 159, 184, 185(photo), 191–92, 256(table); biological classification, 84–85; *Dermacentor* genus, 83(photo), 85, 95, 96, 132, 146, 256(table) (*see also* Rocky Mountain spotted fever); history, 83–84; hosts (*see* deer; mice); increasing numbers, 151, 155; nomenclature, 117, 145–46; and population patterns, 98. See also *Ixodes* genus; *Ixodes scapularis;* tick bites; tick-borne diseases

treatment of LD: and coinfection, 184–86; conventional vs. alternative camps, 79–80, 194–97, 204–11, 212–14, 220, 244–45; costs, 211, 213, 239; Yale team's recommendations, 80, 110, 116. *See also* antibiotics; malariatherapy

typhus fever, 88–89

ulcers, 35, 113–14, 203–4

vaccines: history, 225–29, 235; LD vaccines, 229–30, 231–37, 249

vectors of disease, 42–44, 88–89, 117. *See also* mosquitoes; *headings beginning with* tick; *specific diseases*

viruses, 42–44, 63; suspected as LD cause, 44, 75–76, 126–28

Wagner von Jauregg, Julius, 216–18

Walker, Craig and Mary (father and daughter), 214, 218–19, 220

Warren, J. Robin, 113–14

Watson, James, 221–22

Weber, Klaus, 71, 124(photo), 124–26, 138, 142–43, 146–47, 248

Western blot (immunoblot) test, 170, 175–78, 237

The Widening Circle (Murray), 81. *See also* Murray, Polly and family

Wolfe, Sidney, 234–35

wood tick (*D. andersoni*), 95, 146

Yale team's investigation: antibiotic trials, 110–12, 115–16; bias, 73–75; case definition, 37; causal organism sought, 44, 75–76, 118–20, 123; evaluation protocol, 37, 38(fig.); initial study, 36–45; and the international symposium, 141–43; investigative methods, 37–39, 76, 87–88; LD spirochete isolated, 138; summer of 1976, 75–80, 82–83; ticks suspected, 81–83, 87–88; treatment guidelines, 79–80, 110, 116. *See also* investigation of LD; Malawista, Stephen; Snydman, David; Steere, Allen

Zinsser, Hans, 88–89